Ann Holdway started her training for kinesiology in the late 70's, following on with a course, in the United States, to become a qualified Touch for Health instructor. She also helped to form the British Touch for Health Association, serving on the committee for ten years in various capacities. Before working for a London borough as Head of Sports Development during the '90's, Ann ran her own health & beauty salon whilst teaching and lecturing in the field of health, fitness, exercise, beauty and kinesiology.

'Health Essentials' series

There is a growing number of people who find themselves attracted to holistic or alternative therapies and natural approaches to maintaining optimum health and vitality. The 'Health Essentials' series will help the newcomer by presenting high-quality introductions to all the main complementary health subjects. Each book presents all the essential information on a particular therapy, explaining what it is, how it works and what it can do for the reader. Advice is also given, where possible, on how to begin using the therapy at home, together with comprehensive lists of courses and classes available worldwide.

The 'Health Essentials' series titles are all written by practising experts in their fields. Exceptionally clear and concise, each text is supported by attractive and helpful illustrations.

Books in the series:

Acupressure, Jon Sandifer
Acupuncture, Peter Mole
Chinese Medicine, Tom Williams
Hydrotherapy, Leon Chaitow
Self-Hypnosis, Elaine Sheehan
Natural Beauty, Sidra Shaukat
Spiritual Healing, Jack Angelo

Health Essentials

KINESIOLOGY

Muscle testing and energy balance

ANN HOLDWAY

vega

First published by Element Books Ltd. 1995

ISBN 1-84333-075-X

A catalogue record for this book is available from the British Library

Published in 2002 by
Vega
64 Brewery Road
London, N7 9NT

A member of **Chrysalis** Books plc

Visit our website at www.chrysalisbooks.co.uk

Printed in Great Britain
by Butler & Tanner Ltd, Frome and London

Note from the Publisher:
The books in this series are intended for information and guidance only. They are not intended to replace professional advice, and readers are strongly urged to consult an experienced practitioner for a proper diagnosis or assessment before trying any of the treatments outlined.

Contents

Acknowledgements

I WOULD LIKE to acknowledge Dr George Goodheart DC, the creator of Applied Kinesiology. My special thanks and appreciation go to John F. Thie for having the vision, wisdom and courage to share this knowledge, through Touch for Health, with non-professionals. Without his insight kinesiology would not have grown so fast, expanded to cover so many different branches, nor would thousands of people worldwide have benefited. My thanks go to Katrina Duncan for her support and expertise in reading the manuscript. And also to all the practitioners who kindly contributed valuable information to this book.

Introduction

I FIRST SAW kinesiology demonstrated back in 1977. What stopped me in my tracks was how immediate it was. The demonstrator, through a process I came to know as muscle testing, communicated with his volunteer's body, found out what was needed, and then, by massaging or just touching different parts of her body, he brought about a change there and then. Being a health and beauty therapist I was *au fait* with bringing about changes that took time and effort, often with the help of creams and lotions, machines, diet or exercise. But to just make contact with another and let their body give you information that could then be used to bring about an immediate change was a totally new concept to me. This was my introduction to kinesiology, and I needed to know more.

I went on to study Touch for Health and work alongside the most active instructor at that time, Brian Butler. Most of our weekends were spent teaching and sharing this information with others. When I first started integrating the techniques I had learned into my work some of my clients declared that I must be a 'witch'! How else could they explain how aches and pains disappeared at a touch, that after one session they could move freely when joints had been stiff for years, or how a muscle suddenly became rock solid when they held a specific food in their mouths? Since those early days kinesiology has developed and grown in a wide diversity of ways and new information is unfolding all the time. For me the magic is still there and every now and then I'll catch myself thinking, 'Hey this stuff really works.'

So what is the magic of kinesiology? Simply that you work with the body's own innate intelligence and its ability to heal itself. The latter is something you experience every time you cut your finger and it starts to heal right away, without you giving it a second thought. Every day we create the life we live. More and more the initiative for finding solutions to problems – be they related to health, relationships or self-development – comes from the individual. Each of us is unique, with a genetic blueprint unlike that of anyone else in the world. The most valid source of information about you, is you. When it comes to issues that involve you, no other 'authority', no matter how well-informed or educated, knows your individual inner truth. Your body holds all the answers as to what works for you. Kinesiology gives you the key to unlock this knowledge. Awareness is the essence. The more you learn about your mind and body, how they work and what is beneficial to you, the easier it becomes to create the life you want. Each person's needs are different. You only have one body to last you a lifetime, you are its protector and its friend, you play the leading role in this never-to-be-repeated living of your life, so find out what works for you. Life is for living, loving and learning and the learning goes on throughout our lives.

Kinesiology is a product of the twentieth century: continuing to break new ground all the time, it is the fastest growing natural health care system in the world. People from office workers to athletes use it in their everyday lives to upgrade their well-being, keep aches and pains at bay, reduce stress, improve their performance and help themselves to better health. It is utilized by doctors, dentists, teachers, sports trainers, chiropractors, herbalists, osteopaths, nutritionists, counsellors and many other natural health care practitioners in their work. This book will introduce you to the world of kinesiology, answer most of your questions, advise you where to go for more information, give you some insight into what kinesiology can help with, explain what to expect from a 'treatment', provide you with an overview of the different branches of kinesiology, and give direction to those of you who want to learn more.

1

What is Kinesiology?

TRADITIONALLY *KINESIOLOGY* (pronounced kin-easy-ology) refers to the study of muscles and movement in the body and is widely used in this context by physical educators, coaches, physiotherapists and fitness specialists. Now, through worldwide use for over thirty years, a new meaning has evolved for the word, which is to describe a natural health system used by therapists based on manual muscle testing. The latter is what this book is all about.

One of the hardest tasks for kinesiologists over the years has been to find a simple and concise answer to the question, 'What is kinesiology?' This is not surprising as kinesiology is very much a 'hands on' therapy and it is far more tangible for the person to feel for themselves what a muscle test is, experience the difference when a change happens, learn how their body is responding to the daily stresses and strains, than it is to provide a string of words to impart the same information. Nevertheless, I will offer you a few descriptions which may answer the question for you:

> Kinesiology is a system which links traditional (Chinese) Oriental ideas of energy flow found in acupuncture and acupressure with Western style muscle testing. The idea is to bring about balance within the body by removing toxins, relieving energy blockages, reducing tension and enhancing the body's natural healing ability.
>
> *Alternative Health Care for Women*
> by Patsy Westcott and Leyardia Black

> The synthesis of techniques involves skills from modern chiropractic, naturopathy, osteopathy and ancient Chinese acupuncture.
>
> *Touch for Health* foreword by Bruce A. J. Dewe MD.

> Kinesiology literally means the study of body movement, it is an holistic approach to balancing the movement and interaction of a person's energy systems. Gentle assessment of muscle response monitors [those areas] where blocks and imbalances are impairing physical, emotional or energetic well-being. The same method can identify factors which may be contributing to such imbalances. The body's natural healing responses are stimulated by attention to reflex and acupressure points and by use of specific body movements and nutritional support. These can lead to increased physical and mental, emotional and spiritual well-being.
>
> Kinesiology Federation (Great Britain)

If that hasn't made it any clearer, read on and the mystery will unfold.

WHERE DID IT ALL COME FROM?

Kinesiology evolved from the innovative and inquiring mind of an American chiropractor, George Goodheart DC. In 1964 Goodheart started to use muscle testing to evaluate the effectiveness of his treatments. He would test a series of muscles before and after a spinal adjustment which gave him valuable feedback on how effective a manipulation was for the condition that he was treating. This also led him to look further into the nature of muscle spasm. One of the recurring problems Goodheart encountered was that when some patients returned to their normal life style their muscle spasm would also return along with the stiffness and pain.

His first insight into the revelation that there were other ways of relieving pain and restoring muscle balance came when he was working on a patient who was suffering from severe pain, whose outer thigh muscle (tensor fascia lata) consistently 'unlocked' (described on page 11) when tested. Out of frustration, whilst thinking what to do next, Goodheart massaged firmly all along the outside of the thigh. Much to his surprise the muscle held its position when retested and the pain disappeared. Excited by this initial success, Goodheart started massaging other 'weak' muscles but was unable to produce the same result. It wasn't until much later on in his research that Goodheart learned that he had rediscovered a strengthening technique (Chapman's reflexes, page 26) associated with the lymphatic system.

The first real breakthrough came when he was testing a shoulder muscle (anterior serratus) of a young man who was having problems keeping his job as a manual worker because his shoulder blade kept 'popping out'. Goodheart found tender spots along the area where the muscle attaches itself to the bones, which he proceeded to massage. What he felt under his fingers were nodules (tiny lumps) which seemed to disappear as he pressed firmly. When he retested, strength had returned to the muscle and it remained firm. Goodheart shared this information with other chiropractors and this method of strengthening muscles became known as *origin and insertion massage.*

Goodheart continued experimenting. He noticed that when muscles became weak, the corresponding muscle (muscle on the opposite side of the body) would be tight and when the weakness was corrected, the other muscles that were tight or in spasm relaxed even though they had not been worked on directly. From this he concluded that it wasn't the muscle in spasm that caused the problem but the 'weak' muscle which caused other muscles to become over-tight or strained. One analogy for this is to think of a swing door held in place by two springs; as long as there is equal tension everything works well. When you push the door open, one spring gives as the other compacts and then the door swings back to its normal position. If, however, one spring becomes loose, the opposing spring tightens, tangles up and the door no longer swings freely. Oiling or working on the knotted spring will not rebalance the system. You will have to replace or strengthen the weak spring to restore balance.

And so it is with muscles. For each movement a muscle makes there is another muscle or group of muscles which is involved with that movement, one muscle contracting and the other relaxing. If you rest your hand on the table and tap your fingers you will be able to observe clearly the muscles on either side of the forearm relaxing and contracting in sequence to bring about the movement of your fingers.

This simple finding – that one needed to work on the opposing weak muscle and not the tight muscle to restore balance – was revolutionary. At the time it was common practice to work only on the over-tight painful muscle, using massage to relax the muscle and manipulation if necessary to realign bones; treatment was then considered complete. This temporarily relieved the pain and relaxed the muscle, but the spasm would return because the

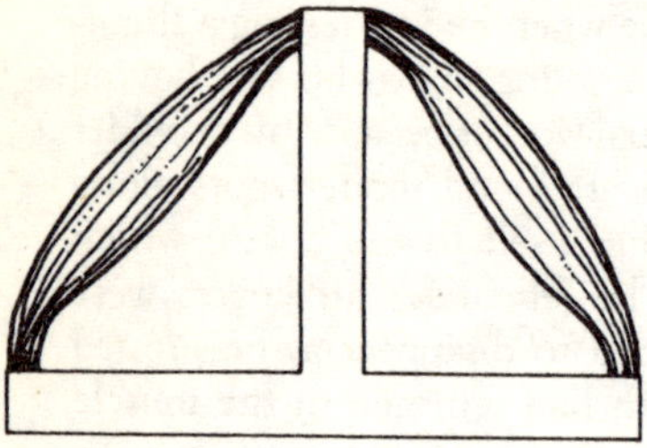

Figure 1. Normal muscle tone

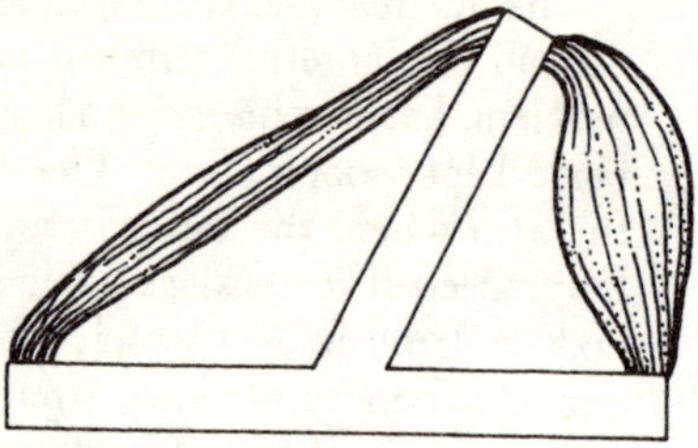

Figure 2. Weak muscle tone causing tension in the opposing muscle

underlying problem of the weak muscle had not been addressed. As a tent needs all the guy ropes to be working equally to sustain a firm structure, so the body needs all the muscles to be performing well to maintain balance. Goodheart had presented us with a new way of working with muscles to relieve pain and tension but as yet he was still unaware of what caused the muscle to weaken in the first place.

Using this premise of working on the 'weak' muscles, Goodheart continued to look for other techniques to restore balance to the body. In 1965 he observed that muscles would strengthen dramatically when seemingly unrelated areas of the body were massaged firmly. These areas were often tender and the tenderness would disappear after the massage. He discovered that these points were part of a wider collection of reflex points (known as Chapman's reflexes and neuro-lymphatic reflexes, page 26) that had been identified by an osteopath, Frank Chapman, and helped to improve the function of the lymphatic system. Goodheart soon realized that these reflexes related to the ones he found quite by accident when working on the man whose fascia lata muscle wouldn't strengthen. This was the beginning of the correlation of various strengthening techniques for the correction of weak muscles which included working with blood flow, nutrition, emotions, meridians, acupuncture points and energy flow.

Goodheart developed this science, shared the knowledge with other chiropractors and demonstrated his findings at seminars, workshops and conventions. He called this new system Applied Kinesiology and founded the International College of Applied Kinesiology (ICAK) in 1973.

THE TRIAD OF HEALTH

Everything we do such as eat, think, walk, fall, is being recorded and has an effect throughout the body. If you have a pain in one leg you shift your body weight to help relieve the pain, thus placing greater strain on all the muscles in the other leg and foot which, in turn, alters your posture and centre of gravity. This, in turn, will create locked joints and pinched blood vessels which will restrict the flow of blood, thus affecting the supply of nutrients to the organs and altering the production of hormones. This means your chemical balance is now changed which affects the individual cells in your body. As you start to feel and think differently you will assume yet another posture, then there will be one more tight area, another pain, one more cycle.

The body is all one interacting unit, an intrinsic whole with many different parts, systems and functions which interconnect and affect each other. Some of the things we do can cause an imbalance in our bodies. The body often sends out warning signals that all is not well, aches and pains, minor digestive upsets, generally feeling tired, tension, lack of concentration, crying for no apparent reason and so on. Unfortunately we don't always heed these warnings and often wait until the body starts to break down before taking any action.

Everything we do has an effect on the body as a whole. This is why kinesiology, like many other complementary therapies, uses the whole person approach and does not look to just address the symptoms. It takes into account the person's emotional, nutritional and physical states and life style, all of which contribute to the overall picture and interact with one another. This interaction means each area is interdependent on the others, therefore a problem in any one aspect can cause disturbances in any other. If only one area is addressed then the problem will not be resolved and is likely to recur. For example, treatment for low back pain might consist of manipulation, spinal adjustments or pain killers. But if that person also consumes ten cups of strong coffee a day which is weakening his psoas muscle (hip stabilizer), is under pressure at work, and has an unsatisfactory home life, then physical treatment alone is unlikely to bring about permanent relief. All of these aspects will need to be addressed for that person to be able to function properly without pain.

A triangle is often used to illustrate the triad of health in

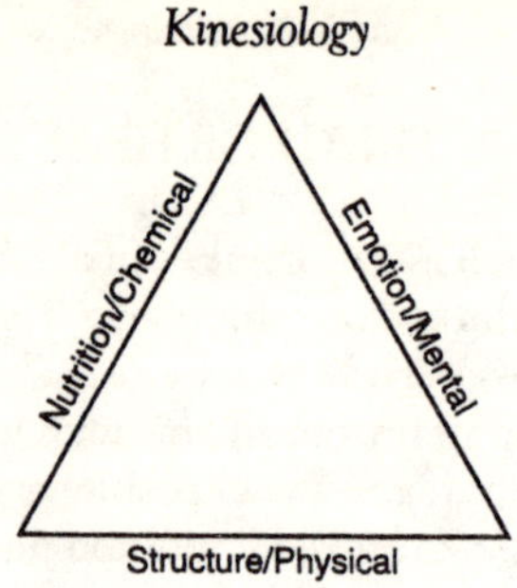

Figure 3. The triad of health

kinesiology, *structure/physical, nutrition/chemical, emotion/mental.* Each aspect can affect the other and we need to work to restore balance between them. Muscle testing can help determine the underlying cause of problems and reveal what is needed to address them.

This is an example showing how an underlying nutritional deficiency can cause a physical imbalance – a connection which would not have been obvious without kinesiology. A client of kinesiologist Michael Kent presented the following problem: his head moved almost constantly and in addition to this every so often would swing dramatically to one side. He had no control over these movements. He was treated kinesiologically with lots of physical work and given manganese to take as his body indicated that it needed this mineral. For five months the symptoms did not improve but at each session muscle testing showed a continuing need for manganese. In the sixth month the client rang to say his head had stopped moving first for an hour, then a whole morning, and since then the problem has not recurred.

WHY TEST MUSCLES?

The body stores the trauma of our lives in muscles and each muscle contains a history of its uses and experiences. Muscles are a part of the body's communications system. Messages are being sent from the muscles to the spinal cord which carries them to the brain where they are received, interpreted and a reply sent which results in some action taking place, all in a minuscule space of time. The action could be a movement in response to a shift in gravity, a change in body temperature, releasing of a hormone, the creation of a feeling and so on. This interaction of communication is going on all the time within our bodies and when we check muscle responses we are tuning into this neurological system.

Picture your body as one big telephone system with the brain as the main exchange and all these messages being transported from the muscles (telephones) along the nervous system (telephone wires) through the vertebrae of the spine (local exchanges) to the main channel (chunk of telephone wires) – the spinal cord. And you know what sometimes happens: crossed lines, calls disconnected, lines permanently engaged, breakdowns, interference on the line. Now it becomes clearer as to why some of our inner messages can also become confused. Muscle testing enables us to tap into the body's communication system, unravel some of those telephone lines when necessary, push the right buttons and help bring the body back into balance.

Muscle Tone, Energy and Function

There are approximately 650 muscles which make up the flesh of the body and account for about half the body weight. Muscles move bones and are attached to bones by tendons. One attachment is the *origin*, which is fixed and the other the *insertion*, which is movable. When a muscle contracts it has the effect of pulling the insertion towards the origin. As described earlier, movement is brought about by the co-ordinated action of pairs of muscles contracting and relaxing. Muscles are always in a state of slight tension – muscle tone – which keeps the body in its upright position and enables the muscles to respond swiftly and spring into action.

Muscle performance is enhanced by the energy from all the body systems flowing freely to that muscle. If the energy is blocked or turned off, the muscle will be working below par. You probably won't be aware of this because the body does its best to compensate for any undue stress and strain that we put on it. Because of its inbuilt ability to self-regulate and correct, it will often cope with the stress and bring itself back into balance. Kinesiology helps fine-tune us when we are out of synch; gives us a set of tools to use to mobilize the body's own self-healing abilities. Like the dial on your radio, if it is a fraction off the correct frequency what you get is gobbledygook; Make a minute adjustment and all the chaos and interference disappears leaving you with clear reception.

> Kinesiology is based on the fact that the body language never lies. Sometimes we do not understand what the body is trying to tell us, but that does not change the fact that the body is constantly expressing externally what is going on internally.
>
> *Balanced Health* foreword by Sheldon Deal, DC, ND

Muscle Testing

Muscle testing is one of the universal tools used in kinesiology, through which the therapist accesses the body's communication system, gathers information on how the person is, acts on the information received and rechecks to see if the treatment has been effective. Retesting the muscle after treatment not only tells the therapist how effective the correction is but also informs the body that a change has taken place – by conveying this information to other muscles it allows them all to adjust to the change. Muscles that have become tight will relax, reset themselves to an appropriate tone and regain postural alignment. When muscles have been given a new message this needs to be reinforced. Old habits are hard to break, as we all know. Retesting anchors the change in the body's systems.

For the assessment, the person lies down on a massage couch fully clothed. Arms and legs are placed in specific positions so as to isolate the muscle as much as possible. Gentle pressure is applied, pushing in the direction that will extend the muscle (take it out of contraction). This pressure is maintained for a couple of seconds and then released. If the muscle cannot hold the position then treatment is given, such as massaging or holding reflex points. The therapist retests the muscle to see if the treatment has been effective. This is part of what is special about kinesiology because you get an answer straight away. Your body tells you 'I'll have some of that as it will help me to work more effectively,' or 'No, that's not what I need.'

Evaluating Muscle Performance

Originally, manual muscle testing was used to evaluate muscle function and strength for the assessment of injuries in insurance claims. This was developed by Kendal, Kendal and Wandsworth in the late 1940s. Various measuring devices were used to gauge the strength of a muscle and the results helped ascertain the amount of compensation due.

The tests themselves are designed to isolate a muscle (or muscle group) as much as possible by putting that muscle in its most contracted position. You can feel this for yourself by placing a hand on the upper chest, whilst your other arm is stretched out at your side at shoulder height. Bring the arm round in front of you so that it forms a right angle with your body; as you do this you will feel the muscle under your hand become shorter and bulkier. This is what happens to a muscle when it contracts. Manual pressure is then applied to see if the arm can hold that position. In kinesiology this is not a measure of strength as such but a measure of the muscle's neurological response and ability to lock.

Muscle testing in kinesiology differs from the original form of muscle testing in three ways:

a. It is not measuring the power or strength of a muscle.

b. It is evaluating the nervous system that controls the muscle's function.

c. The timing of the muscle testing procedure has been changed. Having placed the limb to be tested into the appropriate position, there is a deliberate pause of about two seconds before applying pressure. This gives the body time to record and adjust to the changes that have taken place and to recall previous data stored in the muscle.

What *has* been carried over from those earlier tests are the terms '*weak*' and '*strong*' although this doesn't truly describe what we are looking for when we muscle test nor what is happening to the muscle response. Nevertheless, you will hear the words *weak* and *strong* used throughout kinesiology. Other, perhaps more appropriate, terms used to describe the muscle response are 'switched on', 'switched off,' 'locked' or 'unlocked'. Muscles are turning on and off in your body all the time to bring about movement, following prerecorded patterns that are stored in your brain. Muscle testing uses this binary, on/off, weak/strong, response. The muscles are 'switched on' energy circuits when working or are 'switched off' when efficiency is reduced. You could liken the times when the muscle feels shaky or mushy to the flickering of fluorescent tubes when you are not sure if they are actually going to stay on or not. The trouble often lies with the starter motor. Muscles too need all the nerve fibres to be firing to get a firm 'switched on' response. We are not looking for a contest of strength; what we need to know is can the muscle hold the position whilst pressure is applied.

Tapping into the body's sophisticated communications system through muscle testing enables us to become aware of imbalances. The body does its best to compensate through one muscle for weakness in another. By muscle testing we can ascertain the body's true condition. What we are looking for is a 'lock'. A lock is when a muscle responds by meeting and remaining firm against the pressure being applied. If the muscle being tested feels mushy, shakes or gives way, that indicates that help is needed. Once a muscle weakness has been determined there are a variety of options available to bring it back into balance, some of which will be covered in later chapters.

Accurate muscle testing is an art. It takes time and practice and there are pitfalls. Many of the practitioners in Great Britain started their career in kinesiology through Touch for Health (described in chapter 2), which teaches one how to use all the basic Applied Kinesiology techniques so that you can help yourself, family and friends. This is an excellent grounding for future practitioners because you are learning about your body and experiencing what it feels like. When you later work on clients you are able to relate to what they were experiencing.

Anyone can push on an arm or a leg; there is more to muscle testing than that. It requires a good basic knowledge of muscles, where they are and what they do, proper training and practice. There are many factors that can affect muscle testing and if these are not taken into account then the results will be unreliable. Most practitioners will go through a 'clearing' procedure (page 47) before starting an assessment. Like learning to play a musical instrument, you don't expect to just pick it up and play a tune first time and when you've mastered the skill you still need to tune the instrument before you start to play.

2

Development of Kinesiology

KINESIOLOGY HAS BECOME the general term used to describe the various branches that have evolved since the inception of Applied Kinesiology in 1964. The name Applied Kinesiology refers *only* to the original system developed by George Goodheart and only graduates from the International College of Applied Kinesiology are entitled to use it in reference to their work. Training in Applied Kinesiology is presented throughout the world by diplomats of the college who have been certified as teachers and is taught to professionals with a medical background who are qualified to diagnose.

The methods used in Applied Kinesiology would have remained unknown and unavailable to the majority of the human race but for the foresight of John Thie, one of the early graduates of the college.

TOUCH FOR HEALTH

In the early days of Applied Kinesiology, among the participants who eagerly attended Goodheart's first seminars was a young chiropractor called John Thie. When George Goodheart asked for volunteers for his demonstrations John was first in line. Experiencing for himself the profound changes that were brought about by relatively simple techniques captured John's imagination. He travelled miles to attend more seminars and started using what he learned on his patients with successful results.

After this initial contact, in 1965 John Thie became part of a small group who worked with Goodheart on the development of Applied Kinesiology. In his clinic John began sharing some of the simple exercises and massage points with his patients, encouraging them to work on themselves between treatments which greatly improved their recovery time.

Increasingly John felt that some of this work needed to be shared with the wider population for the benefit of all. Goodheart did not reciprocate; it was his opinion that the techniques should remain with the 'professionals'. Dr Goodheart did however tell John Thie that if he needed a book for the general public then he could write it. John Thie's book called *Touch for Health* was published in 1973. This presented a synthesis of Applied Kinesiology techniques in a form that was accessible and available to everyone. A book was not enough: people wanted to be shown how to muscle test, where to massage, and this demand led to the creation of the Instructors Training Workshop and the setting up of the Touch for Health Foundation.

Touch for Health offered a simple, safe, effective way to maintain health and well-being that was available for people with no previous knowledge of their body or how it worked. John Thie's intention was to empower people to help themselves to better health, not instead of professional care but complementary to it. It is a procedure which allows the lay person to learn the same methods used by health professionals – to evaluate the function and effectiveness of muscles, then, by resetting or balancing muscles, activate the body's natural energies to restore health and harmony.

In those early days one had to travel to America to become a Touch for Health Instructor as I did in 1979. By the early eighties training was available in the South Pacific, Great Britain and Europe. It was this expansion and John Thie's vision of making Touch for Health available to everyone that set kinesiology free. Without this vision kinesiology would not have grown so prolifically.

Touch for Health was never intended to be a therapy. It did however attract a large number of natural health therapists who, like myself, went on to use the procedures with their clients. For others, it was their introduction to health care and it inspired them to take further training and become practitioners. Many of the individuals who learned the effectiveness and power of muscle testing through Touch for Health went on to develop interesting and unique ways of working with it in a wide range of different fields. These new branches are described in chapter 5.

The Touch for Health training programme was expanded further by Dr Bruce Dewe, faculty member and instructor trainer for the South Pacific, covering more advanced information which is now taught in Professional Kinesiology Practice (pages 69–71), and through Sheldon Deal DC.

Sheldon Deal, one of the original graduates of Applied Kinesiology, founder member of the International College of Applied Kinesiology (ICAK) and trustee of the Touch for Health Foundation, shared John Thie's vision of making these techniques available to more people. Since 1980 Sheldon has shared the ongoing developments of Applied Kinesiology with Touch for Health instructors and others trained in kinesiology through his Advanced Kinesiology workshops, which he teaches both here and in America. The developments come from the research papers of the members of the ICAK. Sheldon Deal is head of the board of examiners for the college as well as being editor of its journals.

The International College of Applied Kinesiology and Touch for Health Foundation, two organizations that John Thie helped found, have moved in two distinctly different directions. ICAK moved towards diagnostic and therapeutic intervention. Touch for Health (TFH) continues to provide a self-help programme for the lay person, making information freely available, and does not diagnose, prescribe or treat any named disease. The role of the TFH Foundation has changed in recent years and it is now a research organization. The Instructor Trainers (faculty) and training programme has passed to the newly formed International Kinesiology College based in Switzerland.

APPLIED KINESIOLOGY TODAY

The International College of Applied Kinesiology (ICAK), formed in 1973, provides an academic arena for investigating and propagating Applied Kinesiology findings. As an interdisciplinary organization whose purpose is to coordinate research and educational efforts in the field of Applied Kinesiology, it remains very much the province of the professionals. Chiropractors, osteopaths, dentists, doctors, medical students or persons who have at least four years training in medicine and who are licensed to diagnose can apply for training and membership of the ICAK. The initial training in Applied Kinesiology is one hundred hours long. New developments and research projects are rigorously tested in the field for three years before being accepted as approved material.

Applied Kinesiology is widely used in America by chiropractors and the medical profession. Many Americans visit their chiropractor as we would our GP as their first port of call when they are unwell. Better equipped than the family doctor, many of the preliminary tests (blood samples, X-rays) if needed can be carried out as part of the appointment. Outside the States, Applied Kinesiology is largely unacknowledged by the medical profession. In other countries, the rapid growth of kinesiology has been through natural health care therapists – most of whom would not be qualified to give a medical diagnosis – who recognized the potential and value of kinesiology and began using it in their practice.

Applied Kinesiology is based on the triad of health model (page 8) assessment of a person physically, emotionally and chemically. The Applied Kinesiology practitioner will use muscle testing to find the imbalances in the body, will then choose the optimum correction/therapy, and will later muscle test again to verify whether the treatment has been effective. Examination will include medical history, postural analysis, spinal sublaxations and fixations (misalignment, jamming of the vertebrae of the spine), cerebro-spinal fluid (relates to the movement of the bones in the skull, sacrum and pelvis). These will be combined when necessary with other diagnostic methods including blood and urine tests and X-rays. Coming from a chiropractic background, manipulation and soft tissue corrections will also from part of the treatment. Other widely used corrections relative to Applied Kinesiology and kinesiology in general are described in detail in chapters 4 and 5.

> Man possesses a potential for recovery through the innate intelligence of the human structure. This recovery potential with which he is endowed merely waits for your hand, your heart and your mind to bring it to potential being and allow the recovery to take place, which is man's natural heritage. This benefits man, it benefits you and it benefits our profession.
>
> George Goodheart DC.

TOUCH FOR HEALTH BALANCE

Most people learn about Touch for Health from seeing a demonstration, participating in a workshop, reading the textbook or through a friend and then go on to share these techniques with their family and friends. You either stand or sit to be muscle tested so there is no need for a special couch. The person will usually carry out a fourteen-muscle (one for each meridian) test and balance. This will either take the form of a Fix As You Go balance, correcting any muscle imbalance that is indicated as each of the fourteen muscles are tested; extra muscles may be tested if necessary. Alternatively, s/he will find all the imbalances first, then – using methods related to the meridian flow described in chapter 5 – will look for a pattern which will indicate where to start the balance which often leads to the other imbalances clearing themselves once the main blockage has been released (knock-on effect).

Touch for Health incorporates all the techniques described in chapters 4 and 5 and these can be used effectively and safely by everyone to enhance health and well-being. Through muscle testing you learn from your body what is beneficial and what is harmful to you, the body heals itself, you can tune in and help facilitate that healing process. Working with the responses received from each individual means the treatment is extremely personal and does not rely on previous experience or knowledge. Assessment is being made of the present state of all the body systems – not last week, not tomorrow, but how things are right now.

Currently the emphasis is on the person guiding their own process of balancing, getting someone to push and pull on their arms and legs under their direction. The person being balanced is in charge of the process.

> Every man, woman and child holds the possibility of physical perfection. It rests with each of us to attain it by personal understanding and effort.
>
> F. Matthias Alexander
> (creator of the Alexander Technique)

3

How Can Kinesiology Help?

IT IS NOT an exaggeration to state that everyone can benefit from Kinesiology, acknowledging as it does the individual needs of each person, young, old, fit or ill. It can help with 80 per cent of all health problems that people consult their doctors for: various aches and pains, digestive problems, skin eruptions, nervousness, depression. It can help aid change in attitude, belief systems and behaviour. It can help improve co-ordination, reading, writing, sporting performance and artistic skills. It can help detect food intolerances and nutritional needs, allergies and addictions. How? Because it embodies all aspects of the human being, mind, body and spirit, and supplies the means to improve performance when needed. Kinesiology is not a panacea but it does offer a very precise way of assessing and correcting imbalance. And what is ill health, after all, if not imbalance?

Many of our modern-day problems can be related to our present life styles. In the last hundred years our life styles have changed almost beyond recognition; machines are used to carry out household chores, we eat food that has been refined, processed or treated, chemicals and pesticides are used freely, we ride instead of walking, and watching television is a number one pastime for many people. Our planet is under threat and maybe our bodies too. Antibiotics are prescribed freely from an early age and these are known to kill friendly bacteria that live in our bodies. Will we be equipped to fight off serious infection if needed? Or will our bodies have become so used to all these drugs that they will cease to have the desired effect and our own protective forces will be so depleted that they will be ineffective too? Cases of allergies are increasing rapidly, as are cancer and Aids – all these things are placing increasing burdens on our immune system.

A FORM OF PREVENTIVE MEDICINE

Often we may be unable to prove that having taken certain action has prevented us from becoming ill yet it is obvious that serious illnesses – heart disease, diabetes and so on – do not arise overnight. They are often preceded by a breakdown in healthy function, poor diet, lack of exercise or excessive stress. Discovering unrealized minor imbalances and correcting them decreases the risk of these accumulating and resulting in illness or disease at a later stage. A symptom is a message from the body to alert the person that all is not well. Modern allopathic medicine often uses drugs and surgery to 'cure' symptoms. Complementary medicine emphasises that the body is self-healing and that symptoms are a sign that something is not right and the body is defending itself.

Most of us readily accept the need to service domestic appliances and vehicles as an aid to ensuring they remain in good working condition. Indeed, we are required by law to have the road-worthiness of our cars tested every year. Do we afford our bodies this much attention or do we wait until something starts to go wrong? We often underestimate the wisdom of our body and ignore its needs, yet when the body is out of tune its performance is unreliable, less capable and things soon begin to deteriorate. Reading the self-help chapter, you will find lots of simple ways to work on yourself, and the more you learn about your body the easier it will become to know what kind of help you need and where to go.

A HOLISTIC THERAPY

Kinesiology truly is a holistic therapy, treating as it does the person as a whole, rather than treating symptoms. Kinesiology works with the mind, emotions and spirit as well as the body to improve a person's well-being. With kinesiology you learn to trust the body's own integrity, do not presume to label or diagnose the malfunction and gently encourage the body back to health and balance.

In allopathic medicine, it is likely that if you present the same symptoms as others you will be given the same prescription, remedy or treatment. Kinesiology doesn't focus on symptoms, it asks 'what does this body need?' and often obtains results where other methods have failed. The assessment techniques take the guesswork out of what and how to treat by allowing the body to reveal precisely where the problem is and what is needed to put it in an optimum state to heal itself.

Much of kinesiology's popularity lies in its diversity, for the range of its application is almost infinite. The list that follows is intended to convey some idea of the wide variety of conditions that kinesiology can and has helped:

accident trauma
acne
addictions
allergies
anxiety
arthritis
asthma
attitudes
backache
bed wetting
behavioural problems
bladder problems
breast soreness
breathing difficulties
bursitis
candida
carpal tunnel syndrome
catarrh
chronic fatigue syndrome (ME)
clumsiness
concentration, lack of
co-ordination, poor
cramps
crying for no reason
depression
digestive disorders
dizziness
earache
eating disorders
eczema
elbow pain
emotional strain
eyes
fallen arches
fatigue
fears
food intolerances
frozen shoulder
haemorrhoids
hay fever
headaches
hiatus hernia
high blood pressure
hip problems
hyperactivity
hypoglycaemia
ileocaecal valve syndrome
insomnia
irritability
irritable bowel syndrome
joint pain
knee problems
learning difficulties
low back problems
lumbago
memory, poor
menopause
mental strain

- migraine
- mood swings
- muscular aches and pains
- neck ache
- nightmares
- obesity
- panic attacks
- period pains
- posture
- pre-menstrual tension (PMT)
- prostate problem
- repetitive injury strain
- rheumatism
- sciatica
- self-esteem, poor
- shock
- shoulder pain
- sinusitis
- skin disorders
- sports injuries
- tension
- tinnitus
- tiredness
- vision impairment
- weight problems
- whiplash
- wrist problems

The length of this list may seem incredible. If, however, you perceive that imbalance equals ill health (whether of body, mind or spirit), then correcting that imbalance should lead to good health and balance.

What kinesiology does is to boost and balance the body's own vital life force. It is not the practioner but nature that does the healing, With the support of sound nutrition, adequate rest, nature can enable the body to rid itself of toxins, restore energy flow and release negative stress.

Chapter 4 and 5 contain information on various techniques that may be applied by a professional therapist and in chapter 6 there are suggestions, with illustrations where necessary, of ways in which you can help yourself.

4

Techniques Used in Kinesiology to Balance the Body

OUR MUSCLES OFTEN go out of balance; every new stress we encounter can tip the scales. Think of yourself as an electrical energetic being, with all these messages and pre-recorded instructions being transmitted throughout your body. A deficiency or an excess in this system will lead to a malfunction. When the muscle being tested does not 'lock' (hold that position), it is an indication of an imbalance within your body. Kinesiology tunes into and works with the electrical energy circuits of the body. The treatment methods used in kinesiology restore the energy flow to the body systems, thus bringing about a change. This change is also registered by an improvement in the muscle response – the muscle locks.

The balancing methods described in this chapter form the foundation of corrective treatments in kinesiology. This chapter illustrates how the methods interact and work with the body's systems helping to facilitate the healing process. As human beings we have extraordinary powers of recovery and the body's natural state is to work back towards a state of equilibrium.

ENERGY

The vital force is not enclosed in man, but radiates in and around him like a luminous sphere.

Paracelsus

Vitality, sparkle, zest – this vision of 'get up and go' is what most of us think of as energy, and it is. There's more: energy is not only within us but also surrounds and radiates out from us. You do not stop at your skin: all of us have energy fields, an aura, which goes beyond skin boundaries and can be felt and seen. This kind of energy is referred to as 'subtle energy'. Simply by virtue of the fact that kinesiology is a 'hands on' therapy, through touch we are interacting with the energy field that surrounds us. This interaction of energy fields is clearly illustrated by surrogate testing (pages 45–6), where another person (a substitute) is used to access information for someone who cannot be muscle tested directly, for example a baby or frail elderly person. This method works well for muscle testing plants and animals too.

Everything, from plants, to crystals, to food, to hands, has an energy field. One of the easiest ways to see these energy fields is through Kirlian photography, named after its inventor, a Russian electronics engineer called Semyon Kirlian. It produces photographs by using high frequency electrical currents instead of light. This is achieved by placing a plate between the high frequency current and the subject. A mild tingling may be felt when the current is switched on. The prints show what look like flares radiating out from the subject. Kirlian prints can be 'read' and some kinesiologists have experimented with this by taking a picture before and after a balance with very interesting results.

Kirlian photography could prove invaluable for our health. Research suggests that signs of illness and disease show in our aura long before they can be detected in our physical body. Could Kirlian photography be used to carry out mass health screening?

People have worked with these subtle energies for healing for centuries. The Bible and other ancient literature talks about a person being surrounded by light or light radiating out from their body. Some individuals have a natural ability to see auras, others develop the skill with a little training. The existence of subtle energies is now more widely accepted.

You will already have knowledge and experience of this energy field though you may not have thought of it as energy. You will recall those times that you've walked into a room and have immediately been aware of an 'atmosphere'. Nobody has said anything, you haven't even looked at anyone, yet you can feel it. You are picking up the messages being sent out in the auras.

Remember how uncomfortable you feel when someone stands too close, invading your space without being invited, or the times you've suddenly became acutely aware of someone else, as if you have made contact, touched their very being, their soul.

Most people can feel this human energy field in a more literal sense. Start by holding your hands close together without touching. Take them apart about two inches, slowly bring them back to their original position, then move them about four inches apart. Continue slowly moving your hands back and forth, increasing and decreasing the space between them. Something is building up between your hands. Can you feel it? What does it feel like? Heat, cold, tingling, a pressure: like a force field, there is something there that you cannot see. Once you've experienced your own energy field, try it out with a partner. Place your hand above theirs, palms facing; again experiment with distance. Do both of you feel the same thing? Move your hands over their body, take your time. Sometimes you won't feel anything and your partner will give you valuable feedback on what s/he is experiencing. This three-dimensional energy field or aura is said to contain a record of all your past experiences and your state of health. Healers who have developed the sensitivity are able to see this aura and use their skills to rebalance the subtle energy fields.

As John Thie said, 'All you need is a pair of loving hands.' You have all this energy right there at your fingertips, so you rub here, hold there, and a change happens there and then. Once you know that all this energy is mixing and mingling, it is easier to understand why the change is instantaneous.

BALANCE

In your home you use the thermostat in your central heating to help provide warmth and a constant supply of hot water. Likewise your body uses a variety of devices to help maintain homeostasis – balance: working to keep your temperature at 98.6° (37° centigrade), maintain blood sugar levels and activate homeostasis mechanisms like goose bumps to protect you from hypothermia, fatigue to warn you that you are doing too much and thirst to stop you dehydrating. The word *balance* is also used by kinesiologists to describe what a kinesiology session is and what happens in it. You will hear people talk about *'having a balance,'* *'giving a balance,'* *'being balanced'*. This simply means muscle testing – finding the muscles that are switched off, correcting these with a variety of techniques and restoring the energy flow. Words like *blockages* or *imbalance* may be used to describe why a muscle is not responding and staying locked. When we regain physical, mental and energetic balance, our bodies are able to cope more effectively with all the extra pressures we place on them.

Using the following techniques will bring the body back into balance, by strengthening weak muscles and working on low body energy. They are presented in the order that a lay person would learn to use them. None of them are more important than others; treatment is based on what the body indicates it needs.

BALANCING TECHNIQUES

Nutrition

Food, glorious food. What to eat, what not to eat, too much of this, not enough of that; this will continue to be an ongoing topic with new revolutions taking centre stage every now and then. Most people say they know what they should be eating but they don't always put it into practice.

What you eat and drink plays a big role in how well your body functions. Those of you who own a car wouldn't dream of filling your petrol tank with cooking oil and expect it to perform well. We need to give the same consideration to the food that we put into our mouths to build, repair wear and tear and for conversion into energy and heat. Living in the fast lane, grabbing a sandwich for lunch, rushing to meetings, existing on chips and microwaved processed food, going on a crash diet, all send ripples of distress throughout our systems.

Kinesiology offers specific nutritional support for each muscle which can be used as a guide to what you may be needing. Nutritional needs are very individual and can constantly change. Muscle testing allows the flexibility to meet an individual's varying needs. If the muscle unlocks when tested and the therapist wants to find out if nutrition will help strengthen the body, s/he will ask the client to hold the food, liquid or supplement in their mouth whilst the muscle is retested. If the muscle now locks and stays firm the body is indicating that the nutrition is needed. The reaction is almost instant once the food has mixed with the saliva and been in contact with the mouth.

Kinesiologists believe that there is a reflex action called neuro-lingual (brain tongue), which absorbs food through the tongue and transmits the information to the brain to enable it to assess the effect the substance will have on the body as a whole. This relationship between food and brain is easy to relate to as we know just thinking about something we like to eat makes our mouths water. If the body does not need the nutrition there will be no change in the muscle response. Having looked at this aspect of the triad of health the therapist will then continue to find out what other corrections may be needed to rebalance your body. Placing the food in the body's energy field (pages 23–4) is an alternative to placing the food in the mouth. The food is usually held in the region of the navel or against the cheek.

Reflex Points

The following two kinesiology corrections use reflex points. A reflex is created when treatment to one part of the body affects another part without a visible link. When you press the light switch, a bulb lights up at some distance from the switch. You are aware that there are wires connecting the two points though you cannot actually see them. Thus touching one area can affect another which is at a distance. As you already know, different parts of the body are connected to one another by nerves, blood vessels, meridians. This is how you can treat one seemingly unconnected part of the body by rubbing or touching another part. Hence you can relieve certain headaches by rubbing a specific point on the outside of the thigh.

Neuro-Lymphatic Massage

Frank Chapman DO maintained that stimulating specific points would increase lymphatic drainage in a specific organ and he mapped out these reflexes in 1930. These reflex points are found mainly in the spaces between your rib bones on the front and back of your body; others are on the trunk, legs and arms. They are NOT lymphatic vessels, nodes or glands. These neuro-lymphatic reflexes are points which affect changes in lymph flow.

Our ability to fight off infections and destroy invaders depends mainly on the lymphatic system, which is our protective armed force. The lymphatic system interacts with the circulatory system acting as a filter and drainage network in the body and helping the blood deal with the by-products of cell metabolism. Unlike the blood stream, where the heart pumps the blood round under pressure, movement of lymph is brought about by muscular contraction which pushes lymph along the lymphatic vessels and through the lymph nodes. When the body is fighting infection these nodes can become inflamed and enlarged (swollen glands); the areas most likely to be affected are found in the neck, armpits and groin. Too much fat in the diet can also overload the immune system, making it sluggish and too thick to move along. The lymphatic system consists of lymphatic vessels, lymph nodes or glands, and lymphatic ducts.

Other lymphatic tissue found in the body are the thymus gland, tonsils, adenoids, appendix, the spleen and Peyer's patches which are found in the small intestine. There is twice as much lymph as blood in the body. The lymphatic system produces antibodies and makes the white blood cells (lymphocytes).

In general, stimulation of the neuro-lymphatic reflex points helps the body to 'turn on' the mechanisms which aid lymph flow. Thus it becomes easier to understand why a muscle responds so quickly to stimulation of these points if one has an image of a switch which turns the flow of lymph on or off. It is not the flow of lymph which brings about the change but the 'unblocking' of the communications system which activates a whole series of impulses to allow the body to respond. The lymphatic points occur either alone, in groups, or sometimes scattered over an entire muscle. These reflex points are often tender; the tenderness is usually greater on the front of the body than on the back. These points are stimulated by firm massage, the sort of pressure you use when washing your hair.

Neuro–vascular Holding Points

In the 1930s Dr Terrance Bennett, a chiropractor, discovered locations, mainly on the head, which seem to influence the flow of blood to specific organs and structures. Dr Bennett watched the internal effects of holding these points, using radio-opaque dye and a fluoroscope, a moving X-ray machine. This resulted in both an important contribution to health care and his untimely death from radiation poisoning. These points became known as neuro-vascular reflexes.

George Goodheart found that specific muscles would respond to one reflex only, but that most of the neuro-vascular reflexes influence more than one muscle. In his own work Goodheart found he could improve muscle response by holding these points and he could evaluate that response through muscle testing.

The vascular (circulatory) system is composed of arteries carrying oxygenated blood from the heart to the tissues and veins carrying de-oxygenated blood back to the heart. The blood stream also carries nutrients and water to the tissues, and distributes hormones and enzymes to the organs. It carries away waste products to the organs that excrete them. At any point in time, blood will be involved primarily where activity is taking place. Therefore when you are exercising it will go to muscles, and when your body is digesting food then it will be more active in the organs involved in this digestion. When we are in shock, or under a lot of pressure, we start to lose control. We can't think straight, forget everything, bump into things, don't feel cuts, hit out blindly, don't hear, our vision may become blurred. All of these reactions are brought about because blood has been withdrawn from the thinking part of our brain. Touch can alert the nervous system to our dilemma and refocus the circulation in the body. This is what is happening when the neuro-vascular points are being held, stimulating blood flow to specific muscles, areas of the brain, glands or organs.

Neuro-vascular points are activated by a very light touch. The pads of the fingers are used to make contact, slightly stretch the skin, and are held there. The amount of pressure used is what you would apply if you touched your eye lid with your fingertip. These points are held until a pulse can be felt which has a steady beat. Kinesiologists describe this as a 'capillary pulse', similar to those described by acupuncturists. In the case of bilateral holding points, the pulse beat needs to be felt on both sides and to be synchronized. The length of time they are held can be anything from twenty seconds to ten minutes. There are no hard and fast rules. Remember we are all individuals and our response times will be different.

Holding the neuro-vascular points on the forehead, which are associated with the pectoralis major clavicular muscle (page 35) and emotional stress, will stimulate the flow of blood to the front part of the brain. This will activate the area of the brain that we use when making decisions, thus helping to put us back in control.

Meridians

We can also influence the energy that flows within our bodies in pathways called meridians. Knowledge of the meridian system has been used in acupuncture, for thousands of years by the Chinese to bring about harmony and balance. Meridians are channels which carry the 'Life Force' energy called Chi or Qi (both pronounced chee) in one continuous flow around the body. There are twelve major bilateral meridians which interconnect with each other. Where one meridian ends another begins nearby. There are short connecting channels between each meridian. These meridians have now been mapped out and traced by radioactive dye. Through Goodheart's work, kinesiology is the one modern-day therapy that has added new information to ancient knowledge. This marrying of ancient Chinese medicine and Western anatomy and physiology came about through Goodheart's discovery of a direct relationship between muscles and meridians. He found that certain muscles related to specific meridians. This association of muscles and meridians followed the previously developed theme of muscle/organ or gland relationship. For example, the fascia lata (muscle) associated with the large intestine (organ) is supported by the energy flow in the large intestine meridian.

Chinese physicians (and acupuncturists) detect imbalances in the energy flow by reading pulses on the wrist; kinesiology uses muscle tests to find these same imbalances. When the energy is flowing harmoniously within us we are free from disease. From its inception, acupuncture was thought of as a preventive medicine. People who visited the physician were well and he worked to keep them in good health by balancing the energy flow. If they became ill then the physician hadn't been doing his job and they didn't pay the bill. If treatments nowadays were taken on a more regular basis, minor complaints might never build into major problems as the body would always be kept in optimum condition.

Energy flows through the meridians in a continuous cycle. The Chinese start with the Lung meridian, breath of life. Touch for

Health starts its cycle of balancing with the Stomach meridian. There are two midline meridians which meet where the lips touch: the Central (Conception Vessel) meridian which runs up the front of the body to the bottom lip and the Governing meridian on the back of the body which starts at the tail bone, goes up the spine, over the head to the top lip. These two meridians act as reservoirs and interconnect with all the other meridians.

In Chinese culture everything, including meridians, is classified as being predominantly yin or yang (negative/positive, female/male). Yin meridians are associated with the solid organs (heart, liver, kidneys, spleen) and flow upwards from the earth, yang with hollow organs (gall bladder, stomach, the intestines, lung, bladder) and travel down the body. There needs to be balance between yin and yang for us to be healthy.

When we test a muscle we are also testing the associated meridian and the flow in that meridian. Switched off (weak) muscles are related to under energy in a meridian. The energy flow can be stimulated by tracing meridian pathways in the appropriate direction. Meridian tracing uses the hand's external energy field to encourage the flow of energy in the meridian. The hand does not have to touch the body; working within two inches of the body will still stimulate the flow.

Stimulating the flow in the meridian will also enhance the energy to its related organ. Thus tracing the Stomach meridian (page 34), which starts under the eye and runs down the front of the body to the second toe (next to the big toe), will also enhance the function of the stomach.

Acupressure Holding Points

Each of the meridians has numerous points, some of which have special functions. The acupuncture holding points utilized in kinesiology relate to traditional acupuncture and the Five Elements (pages 38–40). Stimulating these particular points will sedate or tonify meridian energy flow. Acupuncturists use needles, inserted with pin point precision, to stimulate points; kinesiology brings about the same effect by lightly touching the point with the pads of the fingers. Placing two to three fingers on the area ensures that the acupuncture point is covered. Balancing energy with this method involves four acupuncture points, two points being held simultaneously, one on the arm or hand, the other on the lower leg or foot. This means the energy is being moved between three meridians. It is a little like using jump leads on a car where you are transferring energy from one battery to another to kick start the engine. A second set of points are then held, in a sense to close the gate behind you. The first set of points opened the channel, these close the energy flow. Having opened the flow of energy, you also need to turn it off once the energy has been restored to the meridian.

Origin and Insertion Massage

Our heads are held in an upright position by the tension maintained in the neck muscles, despite its natural tendency to tilt forward. That's ten to twelve pounds being supported by these muscles. When you fall asleep in a sitting position the neck muscles relax and the head falls forward. This unexpected stretching of the muscles brings the spindle (nerve) cells into action; they contract, which causes you to raise your head and wake up with a start. This protective reflex action has undoubtedly saved the lives of many a tired driver and wakened many a bored listener at lectures and workshops. Spindle cells lie alongside the muscle cells and are attached to them throughout the muscle so they passively follow the movements of the muscle cells. When the muscle stretches so do the spindle cells. If a muscle stretches too much so as to run the risk of injury, these cells respond by sending a signal to the muscle to contract. This protective mechanism is also known as the stretch reflex.

When a doctor taps the ligament just below the knee cap, the muscle cells stretch. The spindle cells' reaction to this unexpected stretching is to protect the muscle by contracting: this is what makes the knee jerk. The delay between the tap and the kick indicates the amount of time it takes for the nerve impulse to travel from the spindle cell to the spinal cord and back to the muscle. Spindle cells will accept stretching of a muscle when the movement is not too sudden. We can learn a lot by observing animals. Watch a dog or cat stretch. They do it spontaneously, never over-stretching, not too quick, just naturally tuning up the muscles which they are about to use. Fast jerky bouncy movements, especially when used as part of an exercise routine, can bring the spindle cells into action. You can override this protective message, which has told the muscle to contract, causing tiny tears in the muscle fibres. These tears can lead to the formation of scar tissue in the muscle with gradual loss of elasticity. It is a bit like putting the hand brake on in your car for added protection when you park, forgetting about it, and driving off with the hand brake still on.

Golgi tendon organs are also part of the body's protective system. They are found at the end of the muscle. They keep the central nervous system informed of the amount of tension in muscles and guard against over-strain. If the tension is set too high, a message is sent to inhibit the muscle from contracting further as this could lead to fibres being damaged. In kinesiology we influence both these nerve cells (spindle and Golgi tendons) by stimulating them manually with firm massage, working at the ends of the muscle where it is attached to the bone on

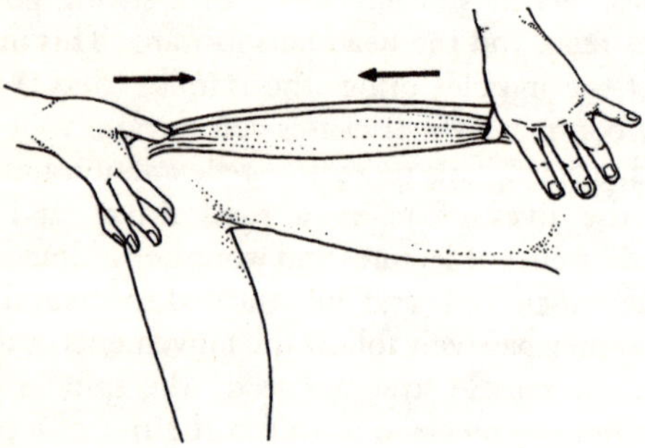

Figure 4. Golgi tendons: to correct a flaccid muscle place a hand at each end of the muscle and push together.

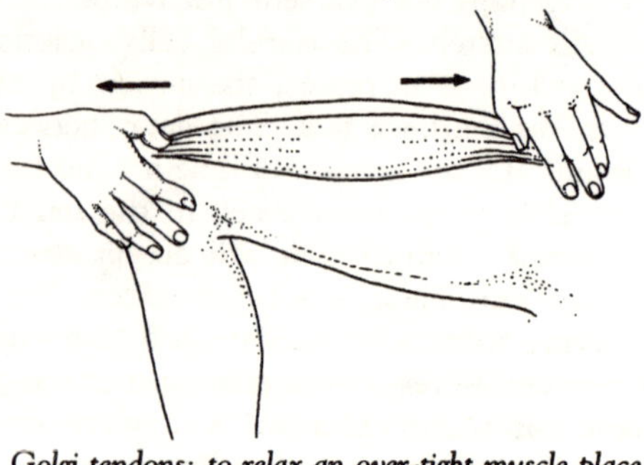

Figure 5. Golgi tendons: to relax an over-tight muscle place a hand at each end of the muscle and pull apart.

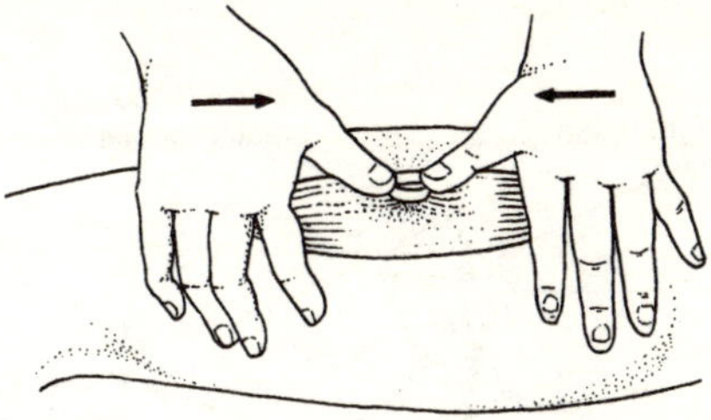

Figure 6. Spindle cells: to switch off a muscle push towards the middle of the muscle.

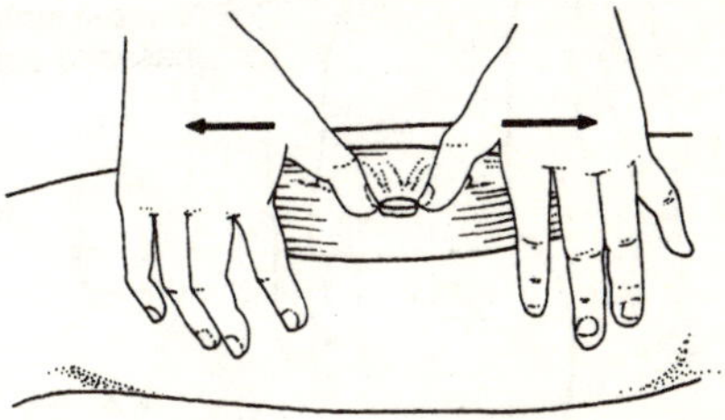

Figure 7. To strengthen a muscle stretch the spindle cells.

the Golgi tendons and in the middle of the muscle for the spindle cells.

This manipulative pressure is used in a variety of ways in kinesiology to treat muscle imbalances. As Goodheart discovered, you can wake up or switch on a muscle by massaging across the muscle ends. To release an over-tight muscle, a hand is placed on each end of the muscle and the action is to pull apart. This action sends the message for the muscle to relax and lengthen. It can be very useful when working with opposing muscles and one is overly tight. Muscle groups work in pairs, one contracting as the other relaxes. If the muscle group that should be relaxing has started out with too much tension in it, this will cause an imbalance in the movement and neither muscle group will be functioning properly. A muscle can also be too long, flaccid. To correct this you need to place a hand at each end of the muscle and push towards the middle, sending the message to contract, This and other techniques which work with the proprioceptors (sensory nerve endings which inform the body about movement and position) are very beneficial to people who participate in sporting activities and exercise classes.

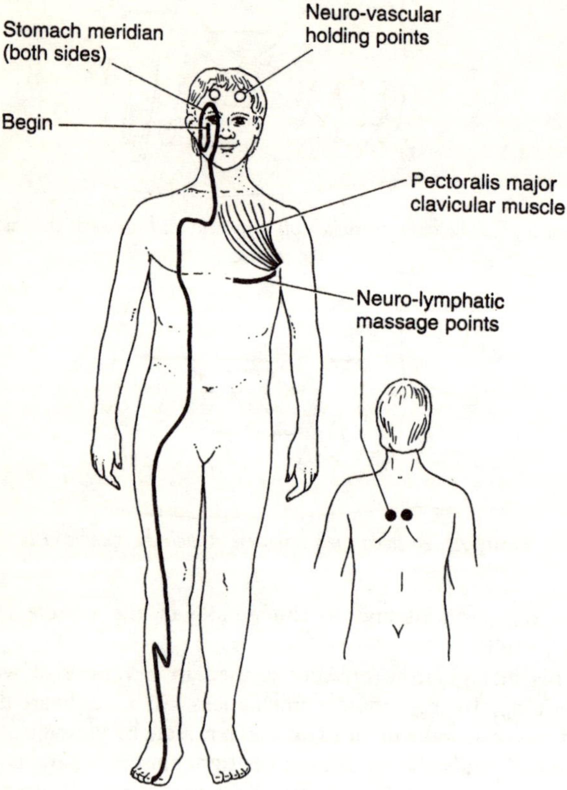

Figure 8a. Strengthening treatments for the Pectoralis Major Clavicular: position of muscle and associated meridian
Figure 8b. The neuro-lymphatic massage points

SUMMARY OF ONE MUSCLE WITH ITS CORRECTION POINTS

Each muscle has its nutritional support, neuro-lymphatic and neuro-vascular points, associated meridian and organ and acupressure holding points. The following describes in detail one muscle and its associated strengthening corrections.

Pectoralis Major Clavicular

Muscle in the upper chest, origin along the collar bone, inserts into the upper arm just below the shoulder.

Nutritional support: vitamin B found in wheat germ, whole grains, liver and brewers yeast.

Neuro-lymphatic points: on the front of the body, left side only, just below the breast (fifth and sixth rib) from the breast bone to the side of the body. And on the back between the shoulder blades about half-way down (fifth and sixth rib) either side of the spine.

Neuro-vascular points: on the forehead half-way between the eyebrows and the hair line. These are also the emotional stress release points.

Associated meridian: the Stomach meridian, which starts under the eye, goes down the face, up the side of the face to the forehead, down over the eye, down the neck, torso, and front of the leg to finish on the second toe, one next to the big toe. The meridian is on both sides of the body and its associated organ is the stomach.

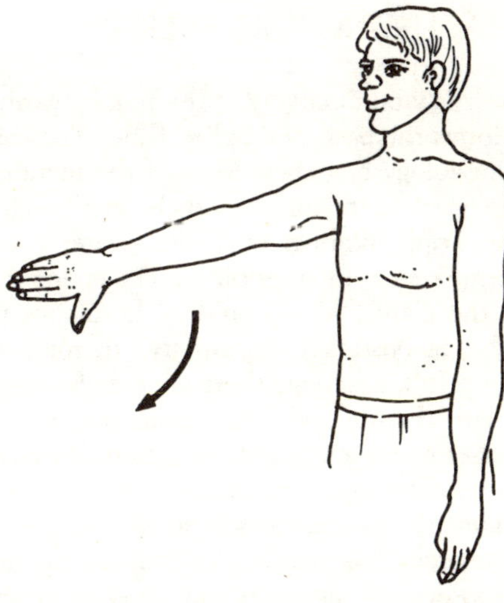

Figure 8c. The muscle test

5

Further Ways of Working with Kinesiology

THIS CHAPTER COVERS some of the other techniques which are widely used throughout kinesiology to ease stress, improve co-ordination and learning ability, reduce pain and discover and correct allergies. It covers in more detail the relationship between kinesiology and meridian energy and how kinesiology uses this energy in balancing the body.

ACUPUNCTURE ENERGY

George Goodheart's vital discovery of the link between muscles and meridians forms the basis of Applied Kinesiology and many of the other kinesiology branches. Most of the meridians have names that are easy to relate to, others may need a little explaining. The Triple Warmer or Three Heater is associated with the endocrine system in kinesiology. The endocrine system is made up of the glands which produce hormones that pass directly into the bloodstream – pituitary, thyroid, adrenals, thymus and so on. In kinesiology there are specific muscles that are associated with thyroid and adrenal function and relate to the Triple Warmer meridian. The Circulation/Sex meridian in kinesiology is also known as the Heart Protector, Heart Governor or the Pericardium. If the muscle test shows there is a lack of energy in that muscle this would also indicate an imbalance in the muscle's associated meridian and gland or organ. Thus, restoring the flow of energy benefits all three – muscle, meridian and gland or organ. The meridian system works closely with and influences the central and peripheral nervous system, therefore stimulation of acupuncture points produces changes both in the meridian energy and the nervous system.

The following methods explore in more detail how kinesiology works with the acupuncture system to bring about balance.

Midday/Midnight Law

Throughout a twenty-four hour cycle each meridian has a time when its energy flow is at its highest and conversely a time when it is at its lowest. For example, the Lung meridian has its highest energy flow between 3 and 5 am and its lowest twelve hours later between 3 and 5 pm. This may explain why some people experience different levels of energy during a day, times when they are at their best and times when they lack vitality. People often describe themselves as a 'morning person' or a 'night owl'. These high or low periods of meridian energy may be the times when symptoms occur. For example, for an individual who consistently awakens with a headache at 2am, looking at the Liver meridian (high energy 3–5am) or Small Intestine (low energy 3–5pm) could provide valuable insights that may help the therapist to decide the most appropriate treatment. Midday/Midnight Law refers to the opposing relationship of meridians in this circulation of energy.

Over-energy in the Meridians

Energy imbalances in the body can be either deficient or excess. What has been covered so far in this book refers to under-energy and the strengthening of weak muscles. A strong indicator muscle (pages 46–7) is used to detect over-energy in the meridians. This time the therapist is looking for a change in the muscle response, for the muscle to unlock, which indicates over-energy in a meridian.

The methods used in kinesiology to detect over-energy in the body involve the alarm points and the acupuncture pulses. There are six different pulses on each wrist on the radial artery, thumb side of wrist, which represent the twelve bilateral meridians. Reading/feeling these Chinese pulses is the most important medium of diagnosis for acupuncturists and requires a considerable amount of skill. The acupuncturist is not only feeling the pulse but also reading the quality of each pulse and looking for subtle differences. This provides information as to any imbalance or disharmony in the meridians which forms part of the overall picture for diagnosis and treatment.

With muscle testing we check three meridians with light touch, then three with deep touch on each wrist. Kinesiology uses the pulses to identify over-energy in the meridians and detects the differences in the pulses through changes in the muscle response. The therapist will choose a leg muscle, usually the quadriceps (big muscle on the front of the thigh), for the testing. The person being tested is directed to touch the area on their wrist where the pulses are, first with a light touch then with a deeper pressure as the therapist tests the muscle. The muscle going weak (turning off) indicates over-energy, which is then corrected by the therapist holding the 'sedating' acupuncture points for the meridian which showed over-energy.

Having too much energy may sound quite desirable to some of us; however, the mother of a hyperactive child may not agree. We all know what could happen if we overload an electrical outlet with too many connections – eventually something has to give. We need to be working on a fairly even keel to enable our bodies to function effectively.

Five Elements

The theory of the Five Elements has been used in traditional Chinese medicine since 1000 BC. Acupuncturists who work with this theory will seek to perceive how the elements are reflected in the person's character and access the emotional nature of the person/problem which is crucial to bringing about harmony and balance.

The Five Elements are classified as Earth, Metal, Water, Wood and Fire. Each element is associated with a particular season, Fire with summer, Earth with late summer (Indian summer), Metal with autumn, Water with winter and Wood with spring. Each element has its own associated colour, sound, emotion, smell, taste, sense, tissues, orifices, climate, planet, compass direction and characteristic facility. In Chinese medicine the five elements represent the cycles of the earth as stages in life: Wood is birth, Fire is growth, Earth is maturity, Metal is decay and Water is death and rebirth. Wood is all organic matter, Fire is gases and

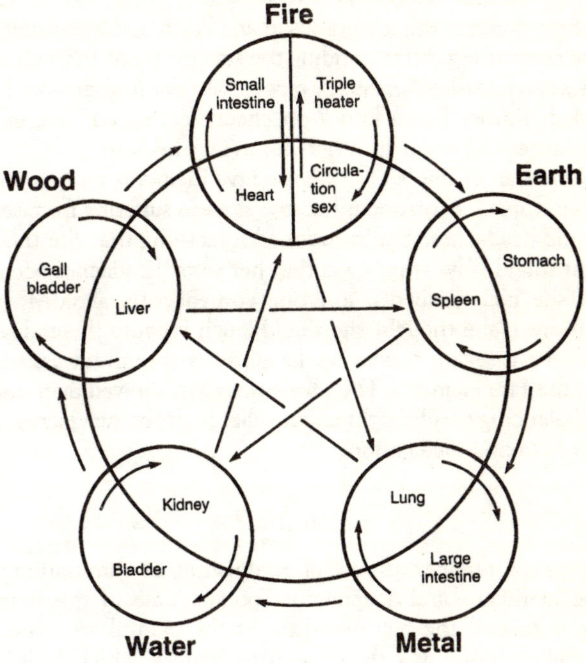

Figure 9. The Five Elements: Shen and Ko cycles

air, Earth is soil, Metal is inorganic matter, fossils, coal, and Water is moisture.

There are two cycles, the Shen and the Ko. The Shen cycle, which is nurturing, generating and creative, moves in a circle clockwise. One element feeds the next: Wood burns and creates Fire which turns to ashes creating Earth; Earth is mined for metals, Metal engenders Water, Water makes Wood grow. This relationship between the elements is described as the mother/son relationship. The Ko cycle represents the control cycle which flows from Water to Fire to Metal to Wood to Earth to Water forming a five-pointed star still moving in a clockwise direction. Water puts out Fire, Fire melts Metal, Metal cuts Wood, Wood breaks up Earth (with its roots), Earth contains Water (ponds, lakes, seas). This cycle relates to the grandmother/grandson relationship, thus if Metal is the mother, Water is the son/grandson and Earth is the grandmother – the controlling factor. Finding the starting point through these cycles can release other energy blocks, without further work being needed. Rather like a knock-on effect, sorting out one energy imbalance may result in others resolving themselves.

Here is an example of using the Five Elements for healing. A woman came for treatment because she was suffering from severe chronic headaches. She mentioned something that she thought might sound silly, which was that her worst headaches occurred after she had laughed a lot. She consequently avoided social occasions if she thought she would laugh because the end result would be a severe headache. Laughter is the sound associated with the Fire element. The Heart meridian showed over-energy and balancing this brought about relief from the headaches after years of taking medication.

Pain Relief

There are a number of ways of diminishing or eliminating pain using meridians and acupuncture points. One of the simplest ways is to find the meridian nearest the painful area and run the meridian one way then the other and see which feels best. Tracing the meridian in 'the best direction' could help alleviate the pain. This method is helpful for injuries, minor cuts and bruises.

Another way of working to clear pain is called meridian walking. The practitioner places a hand gently on the injury, then with two fingers of the other hand moves along the pathway of the meridian nearest to the injury inch by inch. Each time a painful spot is found this is held or massaged gently until the pain disappears. Progress continues along the rest of the meridian clearing all the tender spots. Acupuncturists sometimes feel along a pathway of a meridian to see if there are any tender spots as these may indicate a blockage which can be remedied by putting in a needle.

Another method, pain tapping, works well with long-term and chronic pain. This is an additional technique that can be used after treatment and balancing to disperse any remaining pain. The client will be asked to re-evaluate the degree of pain, move about, perform any action which caused the pain to see if there is any residual pain. If there is, the therapist will then check the acupuncture pulses to find out where the over-energy is. The correction for this is to tap on the first strengthening (tonification) acupuncture holding point for the meridian which is over-energized. This disperses the excess energy and pain.

Tapping of acupuncture points is used in a number of different ways throughout kinesiology. One of the most profound ways works on phobias and was developed by Roger Callahan, a psychologist, who found that phobias related to an improper energy flow in the meridians. He emphasizes the Stomach and Spleen meridians but in some cases other meridians may be affected. Following treatment, the person is immediately relieved of the phobia. The Callahan method of treating phobias is so simple that he presented it in a book for lay people, originally called *The Five Minute Phobia Cure* (now out of print). He has appeared on numerous television shows where he effectively demonstrated the technique with phobias as diverse as fear of snakes to climbing ladders. In seconds or minutes, the person is able to touch the snakes, climb that ladder. Just tapping on these acupuncture points brings about radical changes.

Thought process and beliefs play a major role in influencing what happens in our lives, especially on the subconscious level, and they can sometimes stop us achieving our goals. Callahan calls this syndrome 'psychological reversal'. This could be what is happening when you set yourself a goal which you continually fail to achieve. Some part of you is not ready to take on the responsibility for the success of that goal. So making a positive statement 'I want to lose weight' turns the muscle off and 'I want to stay fat' makes the muscle strong. If the person's true desire is to lose weight then subconsciously there are some fears or discomfort around the issue of losing weight. (This may require some in-depth stress release work.) The correction for psychological reversal is tapping acupuncture points whilst making positive statements. Further description is included in the chapter on self-help (page 67)

STRESS RELEASE

The negative effects of stress (or rather distress), of whatever kind, can be very detrimental to our health. There is a simple yet extremely powerful technique used in kinesiology to release stress. Most of you have been doing it instinctively all your lives. How many times have you held your head in your hands when under stress or put your hands on your forehead when you have been trying to think something through? All you needed to do was hold your hands there a little longer.

The emotional stress release points (see Fig. 11, page 56) are small bumps on your forehead, midway between your eyebrows and your hairline. They are more prominent on some people than on others. These points are part of the neuro-vascular system and relate to the pectoralis major clavicular muscle and the Stomach and Bladder meridian. When the points are held very lightly, pulses may be felt under the fingertips. Initially these will be out of sequence, one beating rapidly, the other intermittent. Whatever the pattern, they will gradually flow together, becoming calm and synchronized, which is a sign that the treatment is complete. Holding these points enhances the blood supply to the front of the brain, restoring activity to the area where we make objective decisions and away from the back brain which relies on old memories and past experiences.

The practitioner does not have to know what the problem is in order to help you; you don't have to verbalize unless you want to. Having found that there is a need to work on the emotional stress, the practitioner will hold the points whilst you go through the problem in your mind. During the treatment you will find your thoughts will start to float away, be harder to hold onto, you will feel relaxed. This is an indication that the process is complete. The practitioner will muscle test to confirm this and continue the session.

Emotional stress release doesn't solve the problem nor take it away. What it does is to put you back in control, without the emotional charge, so you will be able to make changes and find new solutions. You can also use this on yourself. For further information on stress, refer to the self-help chapter, pages 52–6.

ALLERGIES AND SENSITIVITIES

Our bodies are wonderfully adaptable but take time to change. Cases of allergies are rapidly increasing. Whether this is due to an overall decline in our immune system's ability to cope or to the increasing burdens placed on our bodies as a whole is debatable. What isn't questionable is that in recent years we have been exposed to hundreds of new additives, pesticides, chemicals, increased radiation, both natural and artificial, all of which is affecting not only us but also our environment.

Allergies are usually associated with symptoms: rashes, itching, breathing difficulties, runny noses, sore eyes, headaches. Nowadays health professionals recognize that a much wider range of problems, including arthritis, high blood pressure, digestive upsets, behaviour problems, may sometimes be due to an underlying allergy, sensitivity or intolerance. Food sensitivities especially can cause a vast number of physical, emotional and mental problems, well illustrated by hyperactivity, especially in children, and in cases of behaviour or mood changes which have often resulted in violent outcomes. Some people become addicted to the very foods that they are sensitive to, others develop eating disorders. Food sensitivity can also prevent you from losing weight. Common foods that can cause allergic or sensitive reactions are:

Coffee, colas, chocolate, black tea
Tomatoes, green peppers, aubergines, potatoes, tobacco
Dairy products, eggs, mayonnaise
Spices
Salt
Meat, especially red meat
Sugar of all types

Through muscle testing kinesiology can help identify items which may have an adverse or debilitating effect on a person. There are several ways of testing for these sensitivities, some of which are specific to the system of kinesiology that they derive from. Applied Kinesiology and Touch for Health use several muscle tests and, where possible, place the food or liquid in the mouth whilst testing. The person will be balanced first, then the suspect substance will be placed in their mouth and several muscles will be tested. These muscles will be those associated with digestive functions such as pectoralis major clavicular (stomach), latissimus dorsi (spleen/pancreas/sugar metabolism), anterior deltoid (gall bladder/fats). If the substance causes one or more of the muscles to unlock this shows that it is adversely affecting the person at that point in time, therefore abstaining from it for a few weeks could generally improve the health and well-being of the person. When necessary the kinesiologist will carry out further tests to determine whether this is a sensitivity or an allergy. Sometimes the quantity is the problem; a small amount of apple is fine but a whole apple isn't. The kinesiologist will always be looking at the person as a whole and will therefore be able to discover if it is a digestive problem and not the food or even a conditioned response. Some people have convinced themselves that they are allergic to everything.

Take the case of Malcolm who was allergic to a large number of plants. Whenever he came anywhere near any kind of flowers he would sneeze non-stop and his eyes would run. He came to see me one day and started sneezing as soon as he approached a vase of flowers. What he didn't know was that the flowers were made of silk.

Many kinesiologists use kits which contain a wide range of known allergens in glass vials, enabling them to test a number of substances in a short amount of time. Applied Kinesiology requires any substances being tested for allergy or sensitivity to come into contact with the body as it does in everyday life, such as in the mouth, by inhaling or rubbing on the skin. Applied Kinesiology does not accept placing substances in a bottle or vial as adequate. Other areas used for testing are on or below the navel or the cheek. Every substances has its own electro-magnetic (energy) field, thus a substance that would cause an allergic or unfavourable reaction for the person will create disharmony in the body's energy fields which can be read through muscle testing. Putting foods and chemicals in vials does not affect these energy fields.

Health Kinesiology (pages 83–6) has the person touch the allergy test spot, just in front of the ear, and uses an indicator muscle to test the substances which are held against the body just below the navel. Corrections involve tapping specific acupuncture points.

CROSS CRAWL

A practitioner may suggest cross crawl movements. This means moving the opposite arm and leg as you do naturally when walking with your arms swinging freely. These movements help balance and integrate the neurological flow patterns between left and right.

Cross crawl movements use the body to stimulate and balance activities on both sides of the brain. The right side of the body is controlled by the left side of the brain and the left side of the body by the right side of the brain.

Simply marching on the spot will improve your co-ordination, activate your brain, stimulate the flow of lymph, help your memory and concentration, increase IQ, improve your performance and increase your general well-being. Examples of basic cross crawl movement are given in the self-help section. Sometimes the practitioner will combine cross crawl with eye movements, verbal statements, humming or reciting numbers to reprogramme the body and mind.

SURROGATE TESTING

There will be times and situations where it is impossible or impractical to use muscle testing directly on the person. The person could be in a coma, paralysed, have severe pain, speak a different language, have limbs in a plaster cast, or be a baby, small child, or someone who is frail or old. In all these cases a surrogate needs to be used for the muscle testing. It is possible for one person to reflect another person's imbalances whilst they remain in contact.

It is not so difficult to understand how someone else can be used to detect imbalances in another person if we consider all the energy fields that surround us. When we have contact, these energy fields are mixing and reflecting each other. When using high frequency current in beauty therapy, the client and the therapist form an electrical circuit although neither can see or feel this. The treatment involves placing a glass electrode on the client and the electric current can be seen clearly dancing about inside its glass container. If a third party touches either one of them an electric shock will be felt by all three. So the current is flowing from the electrode through both therapist and client forming a circuit although it cannot be seen or felt by either of them. Similarly the surrogate only displays the other person's imbalances whilst there is contact; once the contact is broken, they no longer reflect the other person's muscle responses.

Corrections are carried out on the person with the problem, then the surrogate is retested to see if they have been effective.

The person acting as a surrogate needs to be balanced first to ensure clear messages are obtained. If there is any doubt about the responses during the testing, the therapist will double check by having the surrogate disconnect from the person and will retest the surrogate. The surrogate doesn't usually feel any discomfort during the procedure though very sensitive people may feel changes momentarily within their own bodies. They do not take on all the other person's aches and pains.

Some practitioners routinely use a surrogate in their work, finding that familiarity with the muscle responses of the surrogate makes it easier and quicker to determine imbalances. Also, if the therapist feels the muscle responses are unclear a surrogate could be used to clarify the results. Surrogate muscle testing also works well when testing animals and plants.

DEFINITIONS

Alongside the developments in kinesiology has grown a universal language which is in common use. It will be useful for the reader to have some explanation of the meanings of this terminology as an aid to understanding and for a quick reference point whilst reading this book, attending a workshop, or during a session with a practitioner.

Indicator Muscle

With Applied Kinesiology and Touch for Health, many muscles are used to gain feedback from the body. Increasingly, one muscle only is used to read out the body's responses; when this happen the muscle being used for the testing is referred to as an indicator muscle. It can be any muscle in the body which is performing normally, and its association with a meridian is not important in this context. A 'strong' muscle will show a change in response when that body is subjected to a non-tolerable stimulus.

Muscle Biofeedback Testing

Using muscle testing to access information from the body.

Clearing

All muscles will be able to show a change in response, switch off (page 11), go weak, when appropriate. The ability for a muscle to switch off momentarily is especially important when only one muscle is being used to read the body's responses. The methods used to test this ability in a muscle are: working in the belly of the muscle to push the fibres together (spindle cells, pages 31–3); placing a magnet on the muscle, south pole (on) north pole (off); the person looks at a plus (on), minus (off) sign; yes/no response, person says 'yes' (on), 'no' (off); or making verbal statement 'My name is Ann Holdway' or 'My name is Patty Smith' – the muscle should turn off when the incorrect name is said.

Switching

This is like those times when you can't tell your left from your right; you put your left arm out when you're talking about turning right. This can also happen with the body, when muscles are giving confusing or incorrect feedback. This can be checked through muscle testing and is often included as part of a precheck. The correction for switching and reducing message confusion is to place one hand over the navel and then put the index finger and thumb of the other hand just below the knobby bits on the collar bone either side of the breast bone and rub vigorously.

Dehydration Test

Another precheck test is to muscle test to find out if there is enough water in the body system to enable the muscles to give clear correct responses. We are, after all, made up of 70 per cent water. This is checked by testing a strong indicator muscle (see pages 46–7) whilst gently pulling some hair on the person's head. If the muscle then switches off the person needs to drink some water before the session can proceed. Baldness in the client is overcome by using the eyebrows or some other bodily hair.

Ionization

This relates to breathing in through the nostrils, right nostril positive flow and left nostril negative flow. Both nostrils need to be clear, not clogged, as this affects the balance of ionization which in turn affects the function of the brain hemispheres. Remember how hard it is to think clearly when you have a head cold. The test involves breathing in through one nostril and out through the other, looking for a change in the muscle response to indicate that this is relevant and needs correcting.

Therapy/Circuit Location/Challenge

Finding out which corrections are needed to bring the body back into balance. When a muscle response shows weak the client can, by touching the treatment points that relate to that muscle, find which points will help balance that muscle. Thus the body is indicating what it needs. This same point can be touched after treatment by the patient, known as challenging to see if any other corrections are needed. The person touches the point that has just been treated; if the muscle now goes weak then further treatment is needed. In Applied Kinesiology the patient touching is used to find which treatment will help and afterwards as a measure of its effectiveness and by the practitioner to find the areas that need treatment. The latter will involve a strong muscle weakening when the area involved is touched.

Riddler's Reflexes

These are reflex points on the body and head that are related to nutritional needs. Robert Riddler DC discovered these points and then collated them with blood tests. Many of the points are acupuncture points and when stimulated alleviate certain conditions.

Finger Modes

Developed by Dr Alan Beardall, this is a kind of shorthand for reading the information from the body as it greatly speeds up the process of identifying and treating any imbalances. For those of you who are familiar with computers it is like using the short cuts, control key plus one other key, to carry out a command. The points on the fingers are touched by the thumb whilst the muscle is being tested. Finger modes can be held by either the practitioner or the client and they relate to things like nutrition, structure, emotions, allergy and so on. The questions asked while touching these points are: Is this a nutritional problem? emotional? and so on. New modes are being discovered all the time.

Priority

This is a finger mode which is used to decide if the imbalance that is showing needs to he treated first or is there something else that needs correcting. Often correcting what the body sees as a priority leads to other imbalances being cleared without them having to be worked on directly themselves.

Circuit or Pause Lock

When someone is out of balance there is usually more than one cause or stress and the practitioner needs to collect and retain all this information before carrying out the correction. This method uses terminology that is familiar to electronics and computers, 'pause lock', which means locking the information about a specific problem into the body as a whole. To place an imbalance in pause lock, the person rotates and spreads his legs apart whilst the indicator muscle is being tested. This action transfers the information about the imbalance to the whole body. The body retains this information whilst the treatment is continued. Bringing the legs together will erase the recording.

6

Helping Yourself

A WISE MAN ought to realize that health is his most valuable possession and learn how to treat his illnesses by his own judgment.

Hippocrates

There are many simple, yet powerful, kinesiology techniques that you and I as reasonably healthy humans can safely use to help ourselves. You do not have to know how to muscle test though this may be advantageous if you want to take things further. Many people who have learnt Touch for Health will massage all the lymphatic points or trace the meridians as part of their daily 'health' routine, like brushing their teeth. If you are unwell or have long-standing problems a visit to a practitioner would be best and s/he will also advise you on how to help yourself. If you want to learn more about helping yourself and others you could consider attending a Touch for Health or self-help workshop.

Being able to work to relieve your aches and pains enables you to take responsibility and collaborate with your body to restore well-being. By taking responsibility for your health you are not taking on the role of doctor or therapist but empowering yourself to take care of your greatest asset – the quality of your life.

It was twenty years ago when I first started talking to my clients about the need for them to take more personal responsibility for their well-being because there would be fewer hospitals and less help available in the future. Hospital closures have reached far beyond my expectations, the provision of medical care seems at an all-time low and after-care seems to have vanished altogether. Radical changes in our health care system are still to come. There will always be a demand for medical and professional help and it should be available to all of us when we need it. Learning about your body will help you to be more aware of when you need to seek this help.

You do need to think of your body as a whole and give consideration to what you eat and drink, how much physical activity you do, having adequate sleep and time to relax, learning how to reduce the negative stress in your life by changing thoughts, attitudes and beliefs if necessary. All of these are part of the whole picture. There are numerous small steps that you can take to help yourself that don't take too much effort, like drinking more water.

WATER

Water is vital for all life on earth. It is in many ways a forgotten nutrient although we all recognize it as a major nutrient for plants. Every living cell requires water just as it does nutrients and oxygen. Most kinesiology practitioners will muscle test to check there is sufficient water in your body as part of a precheck (dehydration test described on pages 47–8). There needs to be adequate water in the body to obtain clear messages from the muscles.

We are made up of 70 per cent water. In Touch for Health the recommendation is to drink 1/3 of an ounce for each pound of body weight and to increase this to 2/3 when you are unwell. This means drinking six to eight glasses a day, preferably between meals. Drinking water with your meal dilutes the digestive enzymes making digestion less efficient. And it has to be water – not tea, coffee, fruit juices, colas, fizzy drinks; these cannot be a substitute for water because they are processed by the body as 'foods'.

Thirst is not always a reliable indication of whether or not you need water. A good guide is to have a glass of water whenever you are feeling tired, sluggish, slowing down or finding it hard to concentrate. You will usually find there is an improvement in your ability to perform whatever you were doing. Water is very important to our health. As we grow older we lose our thirst, our bodies dry out physically, shrinking can begin, organs get slightly smaller and so does the brain. Early signs of senility can be reversed by drinking the correct amount of water. Water helps flush out toxins and poisons, slows down the ageing process, diminishes wrinkles by hydrating the skin from the inside and can help you lose weight. Need I say more?

CROSS CRAWL MOVEMENTS

For most of us, life begins with cross crawl as we swim down the birth canal; after the head appears first one shoulder and arm, and then the other. In childhood, if we miss out on one stage of our patterning it could have an effect on our development in other ways later on. Babies usually start to crawl at about eight months and it is during this time that our perception systems are being organized to cross the body's midline. These crawling activities prepare us for reading and writing when our hands, eyes and mind need to move from left to right. Some infants miss out on this crawling stage: they shuffle along on their bottoms or use both their arms to pull their lower body along. Pushing or encouraging a child to walk too soon could also have an adverse effect when the child is older. Dyslexia, cross eyes, stuttering, lack of concentration and clumsiness have all been traced to interference in the normal neurological patterning process. Left and right brain integration is very important for development.

Cross crawl can involve any movements that use the opposite arm and leg. These basic movements are used in kinesiology to help improve co-ordination, reading, writing, concentration, performance in sports activities and so on. The movements themselves involve a crossing of nerve function: this action 'educates' and organizes the nervous system, helping to improve your mental capacity as well as your co-ordination.

Cross crawling is useful before any activity that causes you stress or when you wish to improve your performance such as running in a race or taking an exam. You can repeat the movements about eight times or as many as feels comfortable. Make them part of your exercise regime, smile, put on your favourite music, follow the movements in the diagrams, and you are on your way. When working with infants, it is easier to lay them down and take them through the movements passively.

STRESS RELIEF

'Things are neither good or bad but thinking makes them so.'
Hamlet, William Shakespeare

Stress is a part of living, of being alive, and the right kind of stress can be a good thing as it gives us the impetus to get things done,

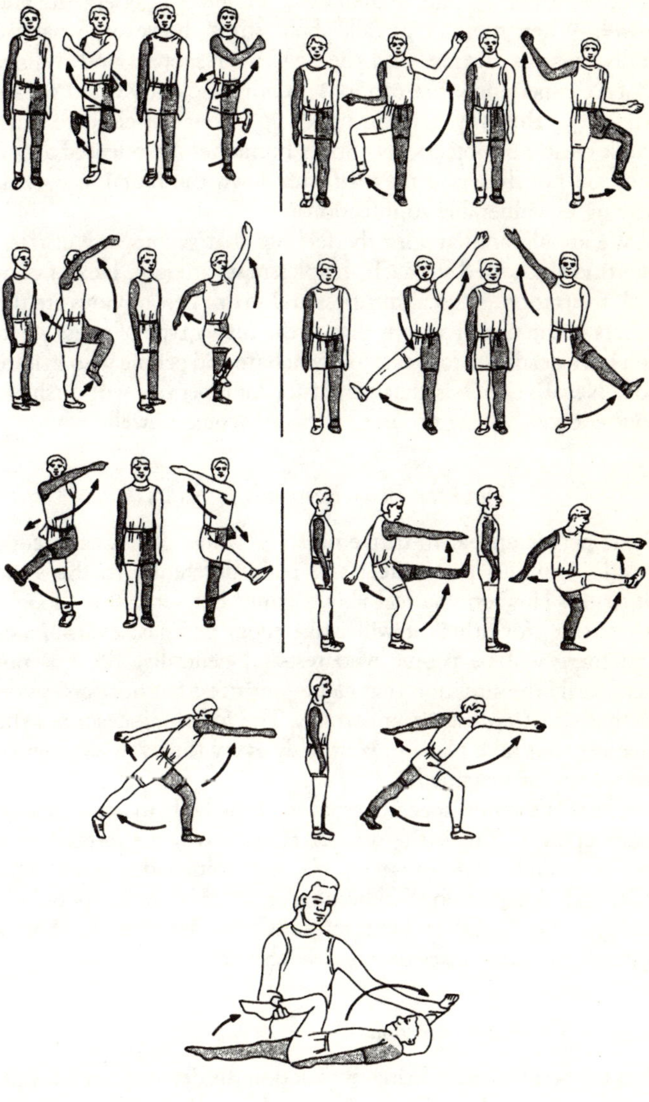

Figure 10. Cross crawl exercise patterns

to move forward, meet the challenges. When we experience positive stress we are exhilarated, stimulated, energetic and joyful. When most of us talk about stress, however, what we really mean is 'distress' and the negative responses and feelings that we experience. We cannot function efficiently when we are stressed in this way; tension builds up in our muscles; we can't think clearly or objectively. Stress hormones are released and if they are not dispersed they will run down the immune system, leaving us vulnerable to infections.

We are all familiar with the feelings that accompany distress: emptiness, knotted stomach, helplessness, anxiety, lack of control, frustration, nausea, dizziness and so on. Less obvious are the effects of the negative daily mood, the niggly type of stress when you have deadlines to meet, jobs you hate and people who irritate you. Negative moods that persist for long periods will dissipate your energy. Sooner or later you will become unwell.

How the Body Responds to Stress

Some people appear to thrive on stress whilst others can't cope at all. And yes, people feel and react differently to the same situation. How do you feel about flying? For some this thought is exciting, for others it will make them nervous, even afraid, and there will be people who respond neutrally. So it is not necessarily the situation that causes our stress but our perception of that situation that is important. The following describes the changes that take place in your body every time you experience stress, real or imagined.

'Stress is the non specific response of the body to any demands made upon it': this is the way Dr Hans Selve, the forefather of stress research, defines stress. He also coined the word GAS (General Adaptation Syndrome) or as it is more popularly known, the 'flight or fight response', to describe the body's physiological responses to stress. These are:

Stage 1: The Alarm Reaction

Puts the body on alert, brings into action the defence mechanism, hormones are released into the bloodstream, arteries constrict, heart beats faster, pulse increases, blood goes from your extremities to your vital organs, skin temperature drops, you lose colour, turn pale or white, digestion slows down, pupils dilate, glucose is released to provide energy. All these changes happen within seconds.

Stage 2: Response Stage

Your body decides what action you need to take. In survival situations you don't have time to think and make conscious decisions, so brain control reverts to back brain where our memories are stored and we react automatically, based on past experiences or information. With the flight or fight response a cat with kittens, if approached by a dog, is much more likely to respond by arching its back, spitting and baring its claws. Whereas without the presence of the kittens the cat's likely response will be to streak off down the alley. In both of these options the stress hormones that have been released will be used up and dispersed. What often happens with us humans is that emotions become involved. We store things up so the stress hormones continue to accrue and the body goes further out of balance.

Stage 3: Overwhelm

The body's prime concern now is to break down the stress hormones. Blood is therefore drawn from the large skeletal muscles in the arms and legs and goes to the abdominal organs. You will be less co-ordinated and become more accident prone. Your brain activity is affected, you can't recall names or where you put things, your mind goes blank. The knowledge is there but you aren't able to recall it during this overwhelm stage. When the blood supply is restored to the frontal lobes of the brain the words will come flooding back.

Stage 4: Recovery

Your body is designed to cope with stress: trouble occurs when the response to stress becomes excessive and your body is unable to dispose of all the extra hormones that have been produced. Therefore the same physiological changes that happened in the alarm stage which were designed to help you, end up working against you if the stress response is being triggered continuously without release or dispersal of the chemical changes. If you are experiencing long-term unresolved stress, the end result will be a breakdown in health.

The Emotional Stress Release Points

There is a simple yet profound technique used throughout kinesiology to clear emotional stress. Start by becoming aware of which situations in your life are likely to stress you. You can then use the emotional stress release points (see also page 42) to help you cope with asking the bank manager for a loan, confronting that difficult person at work, clearing emotional upsets and any other situation where you feel under pressure, not in control or uncomfortable.

Choose a time when you will not be disturbed; make yourself comfortable either sitting or lying down; close your eyes and put your fingertips on the bumps on your forehead, half-way between your eyebrows and hairline. Think about what is stressing you. Keep running the thoughts through your mind until they start to fade away or, if you can feel pulses beneath your fingers, until these synchronize.

Now open your eyes, refocus on what was stressing you, tune into how you feel and notice any changes. You may find you are focusing on a different aspect of the problem and you will need to clear this in exactly the same way. You can also use this technique to create a positive outcome for a past experience or future event. Whilst holding the emotional stress release points,

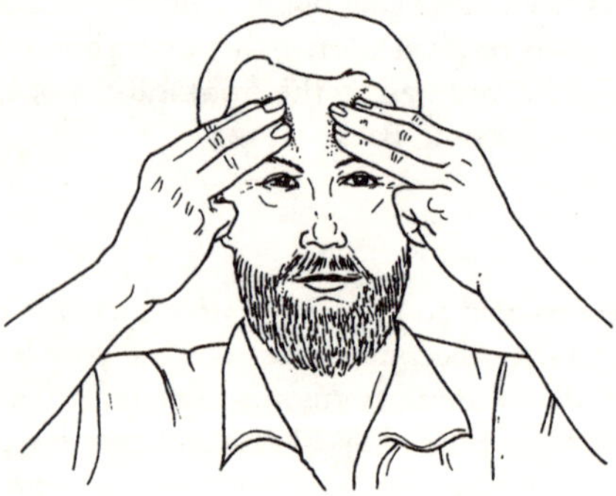

Figure 11. Emotional stress release

run the scenario through your mind as you want it to be. See yourself handling the situation in a way that is comfortable for you and creating the outcome you want. Like watching yourself on a television screen, go through the sequence several times. Use this technique for any situations that you find stressful and for any events where you want to improve your performance. You can use the emotional stress points with your family and friends to help soothe, calm and relax them when stressful or upsetting events occur.

ACHES AND PAINS

Massaging neuro-lymphatic points and other points (see figs 12–15) can help relieve many everyday aches and pains. If you have a persistent problem you may have to look further for the cause and seek professional help.

Low Back Pain

Muscles move bones, bones do not pull muscles. Many of our aches and pains come from postural problems caused by muscle

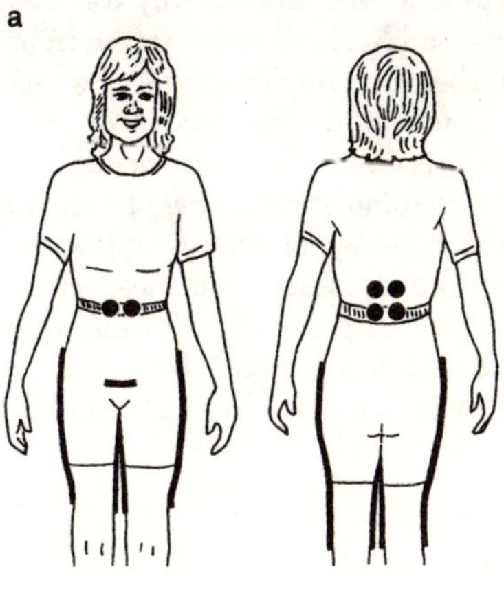

Figures 12a and 12b. Massage points for relief of low back pain: spots and heavy black lines show key areas.

imbalances. It is quite common for hips to be out of line, one higher than the other or twisted forward. An inappropriate structural alignment like this will create an imbalance throughout the body and could create pain in different areas, – low back, shoulders, neck or upper back. Massaging the neuro-lymphatics for the key muscles that support this area may help bring the body back into alignment and ease the pain. Rub these points any time you have low back strain and when you've been lifting or moving things, or gardening. At the front of the body they are located as follows: one inch either side of the navel and one inch above; along the upper edge on the pubic bone; on the inside and outside of the thighs. At the back of the body they can be found either side of the spine just below the rib cage.

Headaches

Nearly everyone gets a headache now and again. For most people headaches are annoying but minor discomforts. For others they can be debilitating, head-splitting nightmares that persist for hours or even days. There are several different types of headaches: migraine, toxic, tension, digestive, visual, sinus. Massaging the following points will help relieve some of these without resorting to taking a pill. If the headaches occur regularly or persist then you will need to look further and ask why you have a headache. Is it stress (mental build-up), physical (tense tight muscles), an allergic reaction, diet, build-up of toxins or what?

The points will often be tender especially if they are relevant, so use firm yet gentle pressure. These are neuro-lymphatic points. Massaging them will stimulate the flow of lymph thus releasing blockages and the build-up of toxins and waste materials. If you are not sure what causes your headaches, reading the brief descriptions may help you decide what kind of headache you have and as you learn more about your body you will become aware of why you get a headache and be able to stop it happening.

Tension Headache

This is the most common type of headache. You'll know the cause; you missed the train, the alarm didn't go off, you are

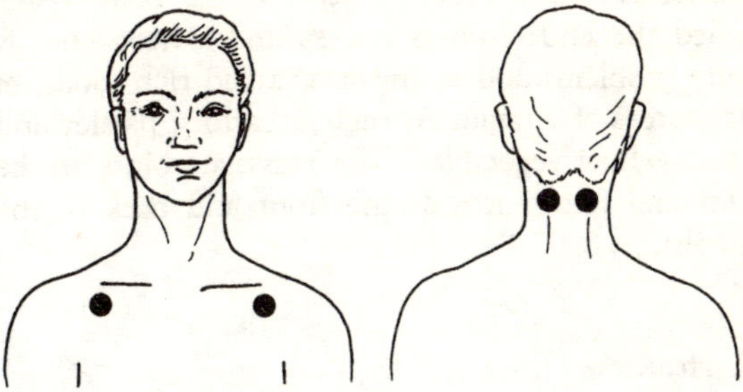

Figure 13a. Tension headache

stuck in traffic and so on. There is a general aching throughout the head and a feeling of tightness along the back of the skull, shoulders and neck. Massaging the points shown in figure 13a helps with all aches and pains in the neck and shoulders, not just with headaches.

Nausea Headaches

This headache occurs from digestive difficulties and correlates very closely with the toxic headache. If the body is having problems with breaking down the food material so that it can be absorbed this could result in the development of toxic

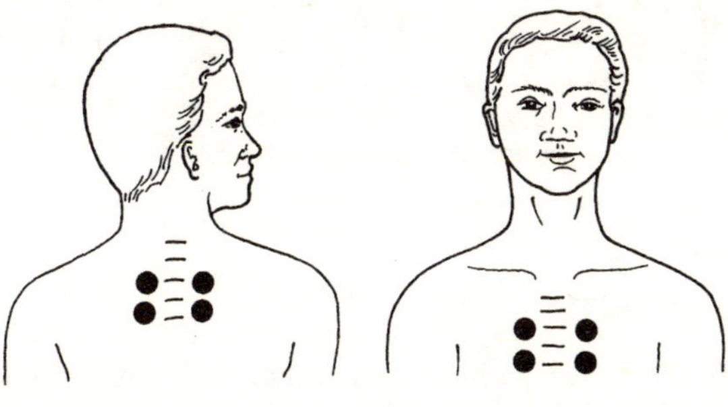

Figure 13b. Nausea headache

food substances in the body. Because the body systems are overloaded the end result is nausea and a headache. Related to dietary problems and eating fats, avoid rich foods, and eat non-fat sources of vitamin A, such as carrots, parsley and other green and yellow vegetables. The massage points are between the third and fourth ribs at the front and back of the body (figure 13b).

Chronic Headache

Could result from overloading the liver. Avoid fried foods, sweets containing fat, alcohol, carbonated drinks and coffee. These neuro-lymphatic points in Touch for Health are associated with migraine headaches. In my experience true migraine headaches will need further help. People who suffer from migraines can often tell when they are about to have one because of the way they feel prior to its onset, and I would suggest massaging these points at this stage to see if it helps to disperse the headache. Otherwise use these points for a very severe headache. They are situated between the fifth and sixth ribs on the right hand side of the body, at back and front (figure 13c).

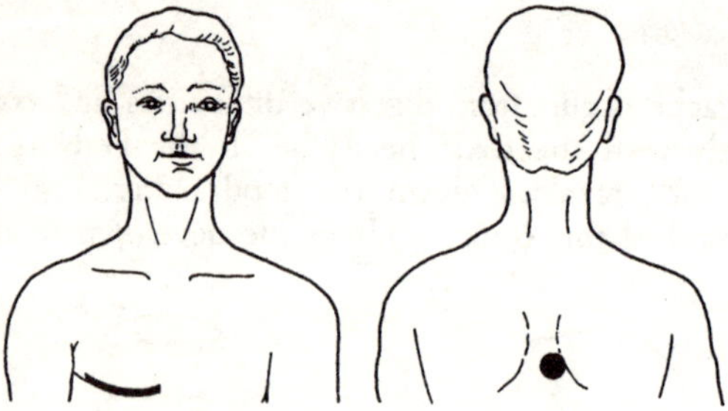

Figure 13c. Chronic headache

Toxic Headache

Possibly associated with nausea, thirst, dark circles under the eyes, shoulder or low back pain, constipation, colitis and other toxic conditions of the body. Can be the result of exposure to

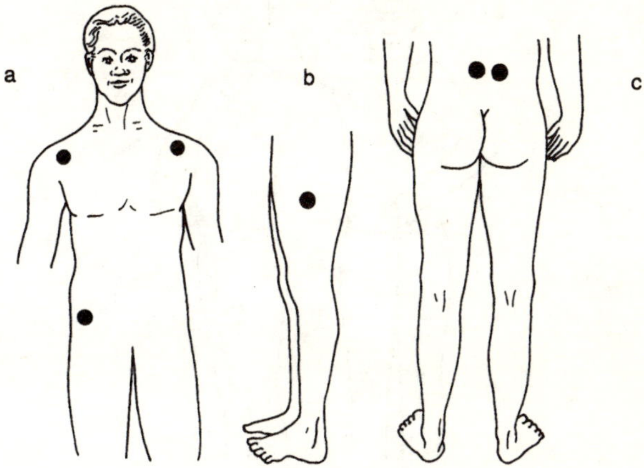

Figures 14a, 14b. and 14c. Toxic headache

some chemical factor, environmental poison like insecticide, household chemicals or chemicals used at work. The chemical causing the headache is usually easy to identify as the headache develops shortly after exposure to it.

What is going on inside your body is harder to identify and it may be related to improper function of the organs involved with elimination, such as the intestines, kidneys and liver. When one of these organs is not functioning correctly this could result in a failure to eliminate all the waste products and a build-up of toxicity can manifest itself in a headache. These toxins are the natural by-products of our everyday foods. Figure 14 shows the massage points. At the front of the body (Figure 14a) they are found on the inside of the shoulders and the top of the iliac crest (hip bone). There is also a point on the side of the leg where the middle finger touches (Figure 14b). At the back of the body there are points just under the rib-cage (Figure 14c).

Pain Release

This technique works for aches and pains anywhere in the body and it comes from *Self Help for Stress and Pain by* Elizabeth and Hamilton Barhydt. First you need to alert the brain by carrying out the movement or action that causes the pain. When you do

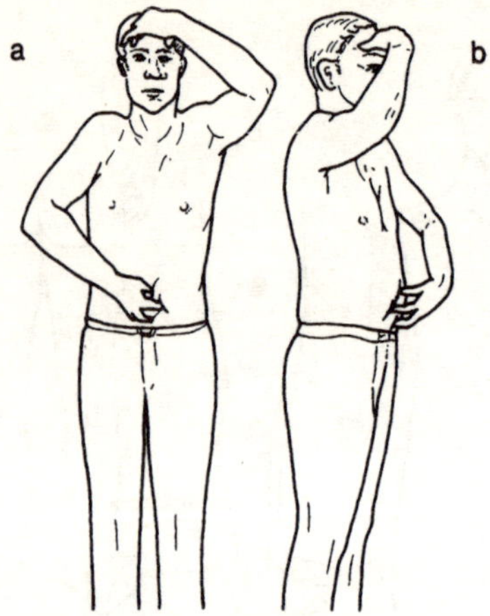

Figures 15a and 15b. Pain release

this it is a good idea to gauge how bad the pain is on a scale of 0 to 10 (0 being no pain and 10 unbearable) as this will help you evaluate any changes that happen.

Place five fingers of one hand around the navel with the thumb directly above the navel. Massage deeply with your fingers and thumb both squeezing and rotating. Make sure your are moving your flesh and not just your clothing; if possible massage on bare skin. It's a bit like kneading dough. At the same time lightly touch the stress release points (page 56) on your forehead.

Repeat this pattern – move the painful area, fingers around navel, massage, hold the emotional stress release points – until the pain has gone. If there is any residual pain it could be because your body needs time to adjust to the changes that have taken place or there may be other aspects that need to be worked on like emotions or frozen muscles.

Treat Your Feet

Feet support us throughout our lives and help keep our balance. Yet they are mainly ignored, often neglected or taken for granted – until they ache. Massaging the points between the toes may help with tiredness and will improve co-ordination when walking and running. Take care as they can be very tender.

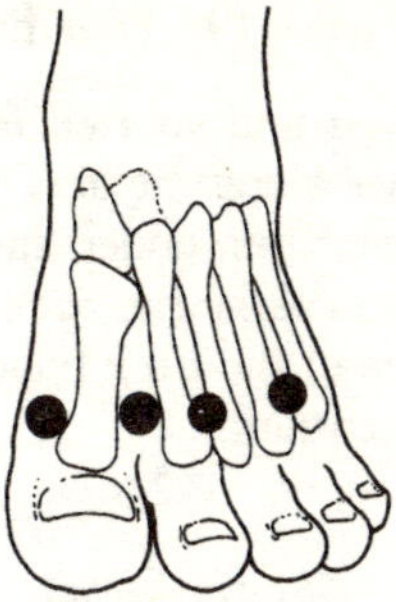

Figure 16. Foot massage points

OTHER TECHNIQUES

Thymus Tap

The thymus is one of the endocrine glands and is involved with the lymphatic system and the immune function. The master gland of the immune system, it lies just below the upper part of the breast bone in the middle of the chest and is responsible for programming all the cells with their own code. This code is recorded and held in the memory bank of the immune system so that the body can recognize its own cells from alien cells. In addition to this, the thymus prepares the T cells for their work which is to recognize friend from foe and to destroy foreign or abnormal cells. For many years the thymus gland was thought to have little or no function in adult life. This assumption came about mainly through the results of post mortems where the gland was usually found to be quite small and atrophied. Now it is known that the thymus reacts dramatically to serious illness and stress and can shrink to half its size in twenty-four hours. The thymus gland's role in immunology is paramount, especially in the fight against cancer. Thymus extract was used as long ago as 1920 for the treatment of cancer. We all have cancer cells in our bodies and the immune system keeps them under control and can destroy them.

Tapping this area will encourage healthy function of your immune system as it stimulates thymus function. Tap on the breast bone where the second rib attaches, just under the knobby bits, using a steady beat or a waltz rhythm for about twenty seconds.

Switch On Your Brain

To wake you up if you find yourself falling asleep at work or whilst driving, massage along the area where the arm joins the body. Work in a curve, from under the collar bone to the side of the body and then massage the back of the head at the base of the skull either side of the neck bones. This will help renew your energy and concentration.

Lazy Eights

Drawing lazy eights helps integrate the two sides of the brain and improves hand writing and other tasks that need hand/eye/brain co-ordination. This exercise enhances the eye's ability to cross the centre of the visual field which is where the two images that the eyes receive fuse and become one. In reading, the left side of the brain identifies the individual syllables or words whilst the right side synthesizes the component parts giving meaning to what is being read. Problems can arise with reading and spelling if the crossing mechanism is blocked, either switched off or receiving distorted messages. Carrying out the following exercises will correct this and improve hand writing, enhance eye/brain co-ordination and may increase memory and concentration.

This exercise involves tracing the shape of the number eight lying on its side, starting in the centre and going up and out. The action of going up and out is required as it is the elementary fine motor skill needed when writing the English language in script form. Work through the following exercises, and, if you

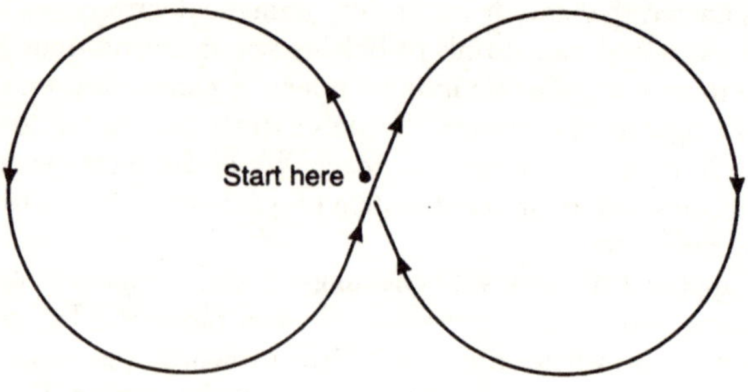

Figure 17a. The lazy eight shape

like, write something before and after the exercises and note any difference.

Tape a piece of paper to the desk, table, wall or flip chart. If you are sitting down make sure you have good upright posture facing the desk or table squarely. Start in the middle, move up and out and trace the lazy eight several times until it flows fluently.

To involve the eyes more, use both hands together with a pen or pencil in each hand. With the arms slightly bent, draw the eights following the motion with your eyes.

Without paper, trace large lazy eights in the air, hands held together, arms straight; follow your thumbs with your eyes. Do these exercises slowly and deliberately making sure your eyes don't skip any area.

Involving more of the body in the movement is activating the main motor skills and different areas of the brain. Whole body movements have the potential to enhance memory, speaking and listening skills. By resting your ear on your shoulder you are incorporating the ears, which helps improve listening and your memory, since memory is largely language-oriented. As before, carry out the movements slowly, use your upper body and move as a single unit.

Stand with feet about shoulder-width apart. Hold one arm out in front, leave the other at your side, raise your shoulder, and tip

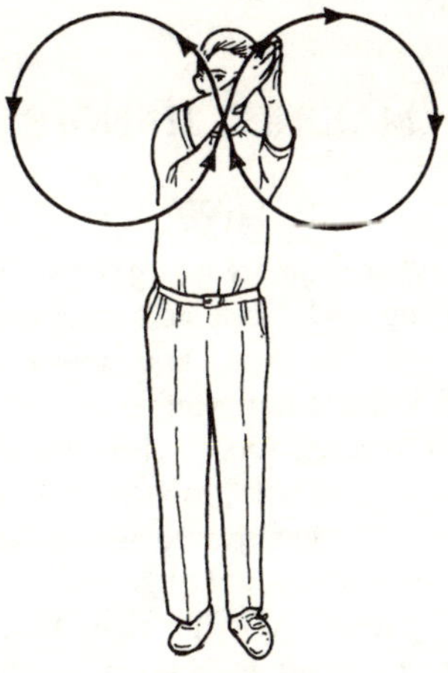

Figure 17b. Lazy eights, with both hands

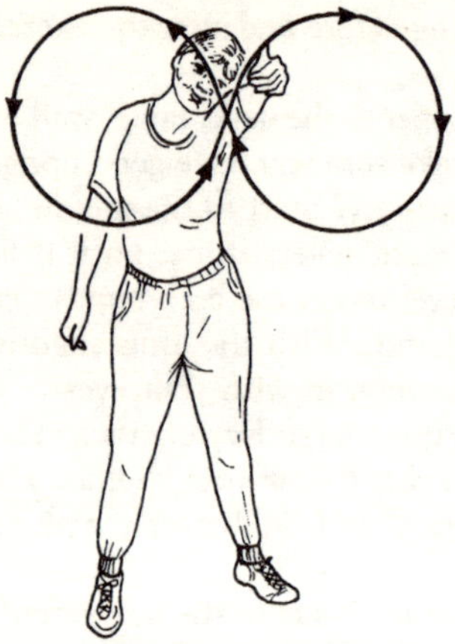

Figure 17c. Lazy eights, with ear on outstretched arm

your head to the side so that the ear is resting on the outstretched arm. Keep your eyes focused on your hand, trace eights in the air, let the motion flow through your entire body, bending your knees to allow freedom of movement and reduce any strain on your lower back. Repeat with other arm. The number of times that you do any of these exercises isn't important; just do what feels right for you.

MAKING CHANGES

Goals

If you don't know where you are going, how will you know when you get there? Setting goals, long and short term, is an excellent way of knowing what you want and how to get it. Goals are solid and you will know when you've arrived because you will have something to look at, touch, show to other people. They aren't set in concrete: they will probably change as you grow and develop. A good way to get started is to take time out, think about all the things you enjoy doing, make a list and see how many of them are part of your life right now. You can go on to write out what you want to achieve in the next week, six months, five years and so on. Support yourself in your goals with visualization, affirmations, use the emotional stress points, talk to friends, read inspirational books, make positive changes and take risks. The following techniques may help when you are finding a goal difficult to achieve. Sometimes there are hidden factors that can conflict with your ultimate desire or you are unconsciously self-sabotaging the results.

Psychological Reversal

Psychological reversal is when your subconscious mind differs from what is consciously being said. The pattern of psychological reversal is seen when you make a positive statement about a goal that you wish to achieve such as 'I want to be healthy', and your previously strong muscle now tests weak showing that some part of you doesn't want to succeed in this. This could be because you think you will lose the extra love and attention you've been given whilst ill or feel there is too much stress involved in being better, returning to work, being more active.

One way of working to change this is to tap on an acupuncture point (Small Intestine 3) which is on the outside of your hand half-way between the base of the little finger and the wrist. Use two to three fingers, whilst making the following statement out loud: 'I profoundly and deeply accept myself and all my problems and shortcomings.' Tap for about twenty seconds.

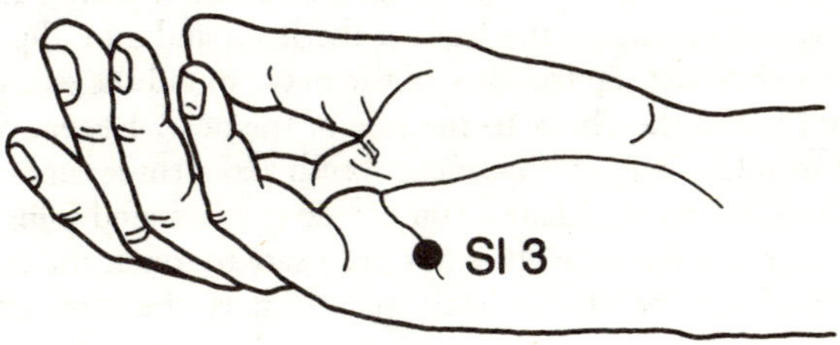

Figure 18. The acupuncture point for psychological reversal

Temporal Tap

This is another technique to assist you with changing habits, attitudes and negative thought patterns. It reinforces any positive change or action that you want to make. The procedure is to tap round the ear, tapping from front to back, whilst making a positive statement. The statements for each ear need to be slightly different. The left side accepts positive statements: 'I always arrive on time', 'I have stopped smoking', and the right negative statements: 'I no longer need to be late', 'I have no need to smoke.' You need both versions to embody both sides of the brain.

Temporal tapping penetrates the filter of the sensory system. The body filters out most of the incoming sensory signals it receives on the basis of 'need to know'. If we were aware of all the noises, smells, touch sensations, vibrations and stimuli in our environment that are going on all the time then the nervous system would probably be overwhelmed. We are aware of our clothes when we first put them on then, unless something happens like we eat too much, we are not consciously aware of them until we take them off. Temporal tapping turns off the filter mechanism temporarily to allow new information to penetrate.

ENERGY BALANCE

This is a simple way to give six of your meridians a boost. Turn your left arm so the palm is facing forward. Place the palm of your right hand on the chest left side of the body, sweep up towards the shoulder and down the inside of the arm. Turn the arm over and come up the back of the hand and arm, dip down over the shoulder, up the back of the neck, round the ear, to the eye and across the cheek to the side of the nose. Repeat on the other arm. Go through this energy brush about three times. This action covers six meridians. You can do it to a friend using both hands at the same time. It is not necessary to touch the person; your hands can be off the body and still have the same effect.

7

Branches of Kinesiology

MOST OF THE branches that evolved over the last decade were developed by people who trained in Touch for Health (TFH) and then went on to combine what they had learned with other specialized knowledge. All of the branches share the same aim of enhancing health and well-being but emphasize different aspects of kinesiology and work in different ways to achieve this goal. This overview will give you some understanding of the different approaches. Some case histories have been included to illustrate further the wide range of problems that kinesiology can help.

PROFESSIONAL KINESIOLOGY PRACTICE (PKP)

This series of workshops was developed by New Zealand kinesiologists Dr Bruce Dewe and his wife Joan. Bruce, a medical doctor, became interested in complementary medicines in the 1970s, discovered Touch for Health in 1977, trained in Applied Kinesiology in 1980 and the following year both he and Joan became instructor trainers for the South Pacific. Professional Kinesiology Practice started its life as advanced information for TFH instructors, who wanted to learn more – the extra skills came from Applied Kinesiology. This early material, formalized as TFH 4 & 5 in 1985, later became the basis of the PKP 1 workshop. It provides a solid foundation for people working as professional health practitioners and, like Touch for Health, does not seek to diagnose, prescribe or treat disease or illness.

Professional Kinesiology Practice introduces the concept of emotions being involved in every problem and works extensively with the emotions from the Five Elements (see pages 38–40). Dr Dewe increased the number of muscles available for balancing by researching the correction points for wrist, hand and foot muscles. PKP has extended the number of finger modes (page 49) available. These have been developed into a 'database' which the practitioner uses to access information from the body. This system allows the practitioner to incorporate knowledge from other kinesiologies and include other natural therapies in the balancing session. The emphasis is on health and harmony and does not balance for the disease process but rather for what the client would be doing if they were free from that condition. For example, if someone has arthritic knees, instead of balancing them 'to ease my arthritic knees' the goal for the balance might be 'I enjoy flexibility and stability as I climb stairs and play bowls' – the two things they can't manage at present. Goal-setting is an integral part of PKP balancing.

Professional Kinesiology Practice, along with Three in One (pages 71–5) and Educational Kinesiology (pages 75–8), are the most widely taught branches of kinesiology.

The PKP Approach

You, as the client, choose a goal for the session – a positive statement of what you wish to achieve as a result of the balance. Muscle tests will then be carried out to determine if this is the right goal for you at this time and the percentage level of stress attached to the goal. A good goal will be stressful to some degree as it will be stretching you, moving you forward to what you want to achieve. The practitioner will then find the emotion involved using the Five Elements: Fire (love, joy, hate), Earth (sympathy, empathy), Metal (guilt, regret), Water (fear, anxiety), Wood (anger, rage, wrath). Then tests and balances for 'Willingness to release the need for the problem' (1–100 per cent), 'Willingness to accept the positive benefits of change' and 'Determination to implement the goal' will be carried out as we subconsciously may be sabotaging our own chances of success. If so this needs to be cleared. Finger modes (page 49) are used to find the priority correction according to the body's responses. You will be balanced in reference to the goal for present, past and future thus helping to clear old patterns. PKP utilizes all the basic corrections previously described in this book and others mainly from Applied Kinesiology. At the end of the session you may be given homework 'to reinforce the changes'. Goal-setting is paramount in this system and as with affirmations the goal is stated as if it is a fact right now. With PKP you are working to balance the life energy forces, therefore a goal for a problem back would not be 'getting rid of my back ache' but rather something like 'I enjoy having more movement and freedom from pain.'

THREE IN ONE CONCEPTS

The Three in One programmes have been developed since 1972 by three exceptional people: Gordon Stokes, previously International Training Director for Touch for Health for more than a decade, who provides insights into the physical, muscle work; Daniel Whiteside, a pioneer in Behavioural Genetics, an academic with a remarkable knowledge of literature and the arts who concentrates on the mental aspect; and Candace Callaway, well versed in metaphysics, who adds depth and insights on where the heart and spirit fit into the programme.

Three in One balances the client on all levels, working with the body, the conscious mind and the subconscious mind, and is especially effective in defusing emotional stress using muscle testing to obtain feedback from the person's subconscious level by asking verbal questions. This involves starting with a switched on muscle and looking for a change in the muscle response. Negative emotions or thoughts will trigger an effect on the body and cause the muscle to switch off; it is this change that the therapist monitors as it indicates that this is an issue and guides the therapist to the next step.

Our beliefs and attitudes are made up from our experience, good or bad, of everything that has happened to us, everything we have ever said, everything that has been said to us. All of this is stored in our subconscious mind and the cells of our body. The memory of past negative experiences is there and has an effect on our present-time decisions even though we may not consciously recall them. When making choices those memories determine our emotional reactions and we base our decisions on how we feel. The Three in One Concepts process works by defusing the negative emotions, freeing you to make different decisions, to benefit from more productive choices and reach your full potential.

Another application of this programme, called One Brain, helps with dyslexia and learning difficulties. It is based on the premise of identifying and defusing the emotional stress from the past which blocked the communication between the different areas of the brain and limited recall.

In spite of the old adage 'Sticks and stones may break my bones but words can never hurt me', words are very powerful. Their effect on both physical and mental performance is generally under-estimated. Words can have a devastating effect on our ability to learn, perform and function. Three in One helps people to overcome the effect of any negative impact caused by opinions and criticisms that they may have accepted in the past.

Three In One Approach: What it Can Help

The Three in One approach can help the following problems:

improving self-esteem
depression, anxiety
addictions
phobias
dyslexia, learning difficulties, poor performance in sports
weight loss

Any problem aggravated by a negative emotional stress can potentially be resolved by this system, which ignores physical illnesses or symptoms, many of which disappear when the underlying stress-related cause is successfully resolved.

Three in One is based on asking the body questions and reading the response through the muscle test. Initially the practitioner will verify that it is appropriate to work with the person before going on with the session. The first step is to identify the unresolved emotional stress and negative beliefs that are stopping the person from reaching their real potential. When working with learning difficulties/dyslexia, Three in One doesn't work directly on the learning problem per se but works on defusing the negative emotions which are inhibiting success, Once the emotions are resolved, increased self-esteem comes naturally, self-image improves and learning difficulties become something of the past.

The Behavioural Barometer Chart

This chart helps the kinesiologist identify emotions that the client may not be aware of. The chart is divided into three levels of awareness – conscious, subconscious and the body. In each of these levels there are lists of words, positive on one side, negative on the other – for example, acceptance/antagonism, attunement/indifference. This approach honours the yin/yang principle, the idea of opposites – light/dark, male/female, heaven/earth – where there is one, there must also be the other. The practitioner uses a indicator muscle to find the primary emotion involved. Once identified, stress-releasing techniques will be used to defuse the negative emotional charge.

Age Recession

Many of our present emotional, behavioural problems stem from our past experiences and traumas. The focus of Three in One is to clear these emotions and memories, thus restoring our ability to make changes and choices freely without the restricting limiting consequences of our past. Kinesiologists can, with the aid of muscle testing, find when the problem first arose. The person does not have to have a conscious memory of the trauma as the memory is stored in the body systems. Age recession, a Three in One concept, is the technique used to find out at what age the problem started. Using an indicator muscle the practitioner checks back from the person's present age (25–20, 20–15, 15–10) and so on until there is a muscle change. Having identified the general period, the process may be continued to pinpoint the exact age when the original experience created the negative self-image. The kinesiologist identifies the kind of energy block or negative emotion attached to that experience, finds the percentage of negative charge 0–10, 10–20 20–30 up to 100 per cent, and carries out treatment to defuse the stress associated with that situation. Having cleared the emotional stress at its source, the person is muscle tested for any remaining emotional charge built up throughout the intervening years to the present time.

Two Case Studies

Janet Bradley trained as a general nurse, midwife and chiropodist and studied reflexology and Touch for Health before becoming a Three in One facilitator and consultant. She has been teaching and practising since 1988.

One of Janet's clients, a man of 31, came to see her because he was starting a new job, he lacked confidence, had previously been told he was dyslexic, was hopeless with figures and had recurring nightmares about his school days. It transpired that at the age of eight he was unable to do his maths for his teacher who, after dismissing the rest of the class, picked him up and threw him against the wall and left him there. This traumatic event, followed by subsequent reinforcement of his difficulties, had contributed to his present state of fear and lack of confidence. By the end of his treatments he had taken a job with a big hotel group, found new confidence and is very happy with his life.

Daphne Clarke, a teacher for over twenty years, now works with kinesiology full-time, helping both children and adults to overcome 'blockages' the Three in One way. She writes:

> A little boy aged six was brought to me because he was unable to speak clearly. He seemed severely handicapped in that his movements were unco-ordinated, his fine motor skills were minimal and he was dreamy, unable to concentrate on anything for more than five minutes at a time.
>
> At his first appointment in July, he was given exercises to help his brain integration as homework; these greatly improved his general co-ordination. We began working on the goal for him 'to learn with ease and to progress'. Used 'One Brain' techniques working on many levels – emotionally and physically to help him achieve hand-eye co-ordination, ease of eye movement needed for reading; release of general stress so he was able to concentrate. By November his parents and teacher were delighted with his progress. He could read and spell words by himself, reading was compatible with his age and his writing was very much improved. He had become a positive, enthusiastic child, instead

of the 'switched off' little boy who previously appeared to have no interest in anything.

EDUCATIONAL KINESIOLOGY

Also known as Edu-K, as the title suggests Educational Kinesiology is based on an educational model rather than a medical, energy-balancing or personal growth model. It emphasizes the interaction that takes place between the brain and the body. As a child you explored the world through the natural development of a series of skills. Thus you learned to roll over, sit up, crawl, walk and talk. Educational Kinesiology uses movements to enhance the learning potential within each of us. All of us have experienced difficulty with some learning process at times, whether it be with numbers or spelling, reading or writing, participating in sports or dancing. Learning breakdowns occur when the information isn't flowing between the different parts of the brain. The movements used in Educational Kinesiology stimulate this flow of information within the brain, restoring our natural ability to learn and function at optimum efficiency.

Paul E. Dennison, Ph.D., creator of Educational Kinesiology, began his search for new ways to help his students improve their reading ability in 1969. His own struggles with learning difficulties as a child gave him clearer insights into how to meet the needs of young readers. Over the next decade Dennison worked with many new and different approaches to awaken the innate patterns of learning that lie within each of us to bring about the desired literary skill, communication or movement. This work included cross crawl movements (page 52), eye dominance, tracking (following an object with your eyes as it moves within your range of vision – similar movements are used by opticians in eye tests) to help visual stress, lazy eights (pages 64–5), and studying how movements affected the learning process. Dennison introduced Applied Kinesiology at his reading centres as part of this study. In 1979 Dr Dennison trained in Touch for Health and began using muscle checking as a teaching and anchoring tool with his students.

Dennison changed his focus from teaching children to teaching adults. He taught his first basic workshop in Edu-Kinesthetics in 1981; the following year he discovered and developed Laterality repatterning (page 77) – a technique which bears his name.

Some of Dennison's techniques and corrections have been modified and integrated into other kinesiology systems.

Educational Kinesiology Approach and What it Can Help

Someone who is:

- dyslexic, unable to read
- hyperactive, can't sit still, fidgets, always on the move
- clumsy, awkward, bumps into things, keeps falling over
- unable to maintain eye/hand co-ordination as in throwing, catching and bouncing a ball
- easily distracted, quickly loses interest, lacks ability to concentrate
- finds school stressful
- has difficulty remembering things even when repeated
- finds it hard to follow instructions
- has poor writing, letters, numbers back to front, writing not spaced, all over the page, slow learner
- confused about left and right
- unable to grasp basic concepts of reading and writing
- drawing immaturely
- reading painfully slowly, full of mistakes, guesses words
- lazy

All of the above are associated to some degree with a learning problem. But Educational Kinesiology is not just for those people with overt learning difficulties. The benefits are just as relevant to those who've never perceived themselves as having learning problems. Educational Kinesiology works to bring about improvement in the ability of the individual to assimilate and recall information which results in an increased capacity to learn. All the parts of your brain need to be working together for you to perform well.

Paul Dennison describes brain functioning in terms of three dimensions:

Laterality is the ability to co-ordinate one side of the brain with the other, especially in the midfield. This skill is fundamental to the ability to read, write and communicate. It is essential for fluid whole body movements, and for the ability to move and think at the same time.

Focus is the ability to co-ordinate the back and front parts of the brain. It is related to participation and comprehension, the ability to act on the details of a situation while keeping a perspective of the self and understanding new information in the context of all previous experience. People without this skill are said to have attention disorders and an inability to comprehend.

Centring is the ability to co-ordinate the top and bottom parts of the brain. This skill is related to feeling and expressing emotions, responding clearly without emotional overlay, being safe, relaxed, grounded and organized.

Laterality Repatterning

Laterality repatterning means taking the body and the brain through a reprogramming process. This repatterning procedure uses a combination of cross crawl movements with visual and auditory involvement which integrates the hemispheres of the brain. When someone has a learning difficulty it means the information is not getting through to the part of the brain where it can be processed and acted on.

The movements used in Educational Kinesiology integrate the brain in these dimensions, allowing information to flow easily from the senses into memory and out again. This enables a person to learn with less stress, express his own creativity and clear the emotional stress that is so frequently associated with learning problems.

Case Study

The following example from David Hubbard shows how Edu-K can be used.

A young lady was in her final year at university, yet her reading age was thirteen, her writing was very poor, not joined up, spelling poor; she was easily distracted and had poor recall, problems with hand/eye co-ordination, always late and confused and hyperactive. She was managing to stay at university through determination and by working extremely hard. Her first balance included the goal 'To keep attention in the lectures and understand the material' and the correcting procedure for this was repatterning. One month later her writing was neater, joined up, and on the line whereas before it had been above or below. She could now copy from the blackboard – previously she had always lost her place – made fewer spelling mistakes, was reading faster, more fluently and with more understanding, and her attention span in lectures had also improved. She continued with Edu-K balances and passed her university exams with grades far above her tutor's expectations.

BIOKINESIOLOGY

In the mid-seventies John Barton formulated a system of kinesiology based on the premise that stressful emotions are the basis of most illness and disease. BioKinesiology links specific emotions and nutritional needs to the tissues of the body (ligaments, tendons, fascia, organs, glands), using an indicator muscle to identify the stressful emotion and its related problem tissue. Correction includes emotional stress release to defuse the stressful emotion, nutrition, and a programme of physical postures called biokinetic exercises Elaborate testing procedures are used to ensure that the nutritional supplement is suitable for the problem and the body as a whole.

STRESS RELEASE

Dr Wayne Topping, a New Zealander, was lecturing in geology at a college in California when he accidentally came in contact with Touch for Health. It was his scepticism that led him to attend a free lecture in Touch for Health after a friend of his had told him that there was a chiropractor who could tell what vitamins and minerals you needed by testing your muscles. Part-way through the lecture the instructor asked for a volunteer with one shoulder higher than the other. No one volunteered. When the participants were asked to stand up so the instructor could pick a suitable candidate, everyone pointed at Wayne Topping. As the instructor worked on him, Wayne experienced changes that he did not really want to acknowledge were happening and at the end of the demonstration his shoulders were level.

It was this incident that launched Wayne Topping into the health field. He studied BioKinesiology extensively with John Barton and is one of the most active BioKinesiology instructors, introducing it to many countries outside the United States where he now lives.

Topping incorporated some of the techniques from Touch

for Health and Applied Kinesiology into this work, added new dimensions to working with stress release and investigated personality traits that can lead to debilitating diseases. Recognizing earlier than most the importance of emotions and their effects on the body and mind, Wayne Topping developed his own series of workshops.

Building on the emotional stress release technique, Wayne included eye rotations, because we reflectively move our eyes in different directions as our brains process the diverse input of information that we receive, as observed in Neuro Linguistic Programming and REM (rapid eye movement) sleep. This involves moving the eye around in a circle whilst holding the emotional stress points on your forehead. This accesses different areas of the brain, auditory, visual, kinesthetic, feelings, helping to remove further emotional blocks.

Wayne Topping also includes eight extra meridians in his work. These relate primarily to the endocrine glands of the brain, pituitary, pineal and hypothalamus, and to the eyes, skin and ears.

Stress Release Approach and What it Can Help

past traumas
sexual abuse
post-trauma stress disorder
stress
life changes
setting goals
reprogramming negative personality traits
defusing emotions

These techniques work essentially on any type of emotionally created problem which can have a physical symptom. For example, many migraine sufferers will have no further migraines after a single session once they have cleared a particular belief that they have internalized since childhood. A case history is taken, clearings tests are carried out, the client is asked what their goal is for the session and tested for priority. This is followed by a fourteen or twenty muscle assessment to ascertain what is happening with the meridian network. The priority meridian is identified and balanced, then positive emotions are worked with using stress release techniques to balance these.

Case Study

The following is an example of Stress Release. One of the participants on a BioKinesiology course had a particular hatred for the area where she lived. So deep were the feelings that there were times when she considered leaving her husband and child just to get away. She begged and pleaded with her husband to move. Finally they found a house and planned to move as soon as possible. Elaine also suffered from allergies which she blamed on where she was living, having never suffered from allergies before. She tried lots of natural remedies to get rid of the allergies but nothing helped. Living in a very small town up in the mountains meant travelling to do any shopping. She hated this too, didn't want to go anywhere but also felt trapped. In the end Elaine went to see a psychologist who, after three sessions, told her the depression she was suffering was due to where she lived and that the only solution was to move.

Elaine asked Wayne Topping not to work on this problem as she didn't want it corrected, she wanted to move. He reasoned it would be much better to move because that was the best thing to do and not out of sheer panic. Elaine went for one session. That evening, after the balance, her husband informed her that they would not be able to move as soon as they thought. Elaine didn't get angry: she found it was no longer an issue, she felt okay about staying.

Next day she had to drive to town which normally left her stressed, uptight and angry, feelings that were quickly picked up by her four-year-old son to the extent that there were times when he would bang on the car windows yelling, 'I hate this car! I hate this car!' Elaine actually found herself enjoying the drive – the green hills fresh with rain, the fluffy clouds in the sky, after seven years. Now she is totally content to stay there and has started planting a garden. All her allergies have disappeared too.

HYPERTON X

Hyperton X is the name given to a system that is designed to identify and release muscles that are in a hypertonic state. Put simply, this means muscles that for one reason or another are in a state of over-tension are not able to relax fully and meet their full range of movement. This can have a profound effect on both mental and physical performance.

Like so many others in the kinesiology movement, Frank Mahoney was looking for answers to his own chronic back pain. First he studied Shiatsu acupressure which led to Touch for Health and he became an instructor in 1981. He was given the opportunity of using the skills he had learned with children who were poor readers, in a junior high school. He worked with groups of ten to fifteen children (forty-seven in total) once or twice a week for two and a half months, spending barely three to five minutes with each child. The results were impressive: some gained one or two years in reading scores, others moved into mainstream classes. It was suggested to Frank that he contact Paul Dennison, as it was obvious that they were doing much the same thing for the simple reason both were applying concepts from Touch for Health. Subsequently Frank joined forces with Dennison, assisting him on workshops and in one-to-one work with learning impaired children.

Mahoney also employs the Sacral Occipital technique, which corrects any mechanical interference between the skull, spine and sacrum (triangular bone at the base of the spine). This is where body/mind integration takes place, sending messages from the body to the brain and vice versa. Working with these new concepts led Frank Mahoney to develop Hyperton X, which deals with hypertonic muscles and tissue that are interfering with the free and proper movement between cranium, spine and sacrum.

Hyperton X Approach and What it Can Help

learning difficulties	accident trauma
sports performance	cerebral palsy
ME	emotional problems
acute and chronic pain	spinal stress
breathing problems	stroke patient
repetitive strain injury	

One of the differences between Hyperton X and the other kinesiologies is that muscles are tested in extension (stretched), taking the muscle to its fullest range of movement and not in a shortened contracted position. Testing is then carried out using an indicator muscle – the test is not carried out directly on the muscle being stretched. If the muscle is hypertonic a series of gentle isometric contractions are used to detect if the muscle will release, stretch further. Isometric contractions occur when two opposing forces meet with enough pressure to remain static, as used in some strengthening exercises. Hence if you place the palms of your hands together in front of you, fingertips to the ceiling, and push with equal strength the muscles in your upper chest will contract.

Hypertonic muscles can be present in the body through any repetitive activity where muscles are used in the same way day in day out, such as working a piece of machinery, hunched over a desk, pushing pedals up and down or using a keyboard. All these repetitive actions can cause tension and tightness to build up in muscles. Athletes who over-train, neglect to warm up or cool down, or don't vary their training routine can be heading for the same problem.

Muscles can also remain in a hypertonic state through injuries – even an injury which has long since healed, if the messages from the nerve cells have become confused or if the emotional aspect of the accident is involved. Mahoney concludes that this overprotection jams the sensory processes, thus stopping the messages getting through.

The symptoms are always restricted range of movement, sometimes pain and weakness. Getting the person to put their body into the position at the time of the accident, testing for hypertonic muscles and releasing them, is a highly effective way of working with this technique. The technique can also be used to improve performance, such as golfer's a swing, tennis strokes, cricket run ups and bowling, by having the person perform the movement and working to release any hypertonic muscles that hinder the free flow of that movement.

Case Studies

A profound example of how old injuries can affect our lives in the present is the case of a patient helped by Joan Brown Rigg, using a mixture of Hyperton X and Stress Release.

A man whose wife had suffered with a pain between her shoulders for some forty years contacted the Bognor Centre for help. The problem had totally ruined their married life, they rarely went anywhere, couldn't plan anything because the only relief his wife got was when she lay down. The lady arrived at the Centre with her arm bent and raised up in the air; this was the only position that gave her a modicum of comfort. A surrogate was used throughout the session, at the end of which the woman could bring her arm down and there was some relief. At a later visit it became apparent that the pain related to a childhood accident around which there were still unresolved emotions. As a young girl she had fallen whilst climbing a tree with some boys; the emotional charge that remained was connected with how she had landed and her resultant embarrassment. Her action to save herself from falling had been to reach up to grab the branch above.

Hilary Marks, a practitioner and teacher of Hyperton X, works with her clients on a very intuitive level, giving them choices in how they would like to be worked on and asking them to create their own symbols for healing. Hilary's present to a girl with lymphoma was that she would work with her once a week or whenever the girl wanted her to. The sessions involved a lot of the spiritual connection aspect from Hyperton X and when asked how she felt this had helped her the girl described it in a form of measurements. All that the doctors and medicine provided represented 12 inches, what she herself had put in plus the support of her family and friends was maybe 8 inches, the spiritual connection gave her 4 extra inches – a focus which pulled everything together. She needed all of these to make it work. The spirituality focus made it real: she felt happier, more positive, had more energy, 'it was the spark that made the bell ring'.

HEALTH KINESIOLOGY

Dr Jimmy Scott is a psychologist and natural healing/nutritional consultant who began working with kinesiology in 1978. He started by using muscle testing with his patients, which he found to be more sensitive and reliable when working with nutrition and allergies than other conventional testing methods. Working with the energy concept from kinesiology he began developing new techniques for identifying and correcting allergies and went on to create a comprehensive powerful structured system which he called Health Kinesiology.

Jimmy Scott sees Health Kinesiology as a whole new approach, a way of thinking and a method of discovery. One of his primary concerns was that the treatments would be 'robust' and that corrections would only have to be done once for each individual. Health Kinesiology is based on the Five Element theory (pages 38–40) and over-energy in the meridians (pages 37–8), working with meridians in very different ways to those used in other kinesiologies. Meridians are coupled, numbered and referred to as elements: Central and Governing element no. 0, Gall Bladder/Liver no. 1, Bladder/Kidney no. 2, Large Intestine/Lung no. 3, Stomach/Spleen no. 4, Triple Warmer/Circulation/Sex no. 5, Small Intestine/Heart no. 6. All the reflex correction points or acupuncture points are just held. It is an a open-ended system not based on a set of corrections for each imbalance, and uses verbal questions working from the premise that the body knows exactly what it needs to bring about a state of healing and wholeness. The strength of Health Kinesiology lies in finding and correcting physical, psychological and environmental stresses. It is concerned not only with the cause of a particular set of symptoms, but also with looking at the process which helps to keep that problem going.

Health Kinesiology Approach and What it Can Help

all physical problems
self-image
lack of confidence
fears
improve sporting performance
allergies
trauma-related conditions
problems particularly concerned with the effect of electrical fields, electromagnetic stress from televisions, computers, micro waves etc
geopathic stress, ley lines

At the start of the session the therapist will ensure that the meridian system is in balance, otherwise accurate information cannot be accessed from the body. An indicator muscle is used for testing and the person being tested places the palm of their hand over the navel, as this area contains reflex points for the

Five Elements. The therapist always checks s/he has permission to work on the person and is looking for what needs to be done, not just the cause, looking at all the facets involved with the problem.

Corrective treatments include the meridian beginning and end points, acupuncture holding points, neuro-lymphatics (page 26), neuro-vasculars (page 27) and sometimes additional sensory materials may be included, such as herbs, gems, essential oils, homoeopathic remedies, magnets, crystals, flower and tree essences. On occasions the person also has to touch a particular area of their body or is asked to think about something specific as part of the correcting process. All the items that are needed are placed on the person's body, all the points are held which may involve the client in holding points too, and the therapist waits for the correction to be completed, which is sometimes indicated by the body relaxing or a sigh or a yawn. The therapist then rechecks that the problem is no longer causing stress. Health Kinesiology acknowledges that for the body to heal itself energy corrections alone may not be sufficient, so it includes analysis and advice on life balance for diet, rest, exercises, affirmations, visualizations, and also addresses the importance of geopathic and environmental stress.

You don't need to be unwell to benefit from Health Kinesiology, correcting imbalances can help you achieve your goals in life. Health Kinesiology has been successful with a wide range of problems, as the following case histories illustrate, and the therapists themselves never know what is going to emerge. Three clients can come in one after the other all suffering from the same PMT symptoms but they will have totally different issues and the corrections will be different too.

Case Histories

Ann Parker, a Health Kinesiology teacher, related what happened to her after attending her first course. Whilst testing a lady who had come about migraine headaches, the response that came from the body as to what needed to be looked at was the left foot. When Ann had taken the client's notes there had been no mention of her left foot so, with some trepidation, Ann asked if there was anything wrong with this foot. She replied, 'Oh yes,

I was born with a clubbed foot.' The client had had fifteen operations between the ages of fourteen and seventeen and had experienced no feeling in that foot from the ankle down for thirty years. Treatment took two sessions and during the second session, when Ann went to hold some points on the left foot, the woman let out a cry. When asked what was the matter she replied, 'I can feel your hands.' The lack of feeling in her left foot had been so profound that on one occasion, when she had kicked off her shoes at a theatre performance, she had walked home in the snow totally unaware that she didn't have her shoe on. This lady no longer has migraine headaches which were partly caused because she walked so badly.

Jane Thurnall-Read is the most experienced Health Kinesiology therapist in the UK, having worked with this system for fourteen years. As well as running a busy practice in Cornwall and seeing clients regularly in London, she is also responsible for the training of other Health Kinesiology practitioners. The following are some of her case studies.

Alice was in her thirties and had suffered from psoriasis for nearly ten years. During one appointment psychological issues to do with hope and love were worked on. Jane used a procedure known as SET to detoxify Alice's body; up to this point her body had been using psoriasis scales as a way of removing toxins. Alice was unable to come back for further appointments. Later that year Jane received a letter from Alice: 'Within six weeks of seeing you, there was a definite decrease in the size of the psoriasis on my trunk. This is the first time in the ten years that I have suffered from psoriasis that it has actually got better apart from sunbathing. I hope that after further treatment with you it might be cleared completely.'

Philip was slowly losing the sight in both his eyes when he consulted Jane. He had previously received laser treatment at an eye hospital but without any real success. He had stopped driving and had become more dependent on other people because of his declining eyesight. Jane worked on the light sensitive receptors in Philip's eyes. By the time of his third appointment he reported that his eyesight was improving and that he was once again able to read a newspaper with his reading glasses. Jane discharged him after three sessions. His eyesight continues to improve, he has gone back to driving a car and taken up wood-turning as a hobby.

KINERGETICS

Kinergetics is a creative, diverse kinesiology system that uses healing energy, channelled through the hands, as the only correction. Developed in 1991 by Philip Rafferty, Kinergetics combines the healing principles of Reiki and Kinesiology. The Kinergetics system accesses the energetic imbalances and blockages which are the cause of all physical symptoms, and then directs healing energy where the body itself has indicated, allowing the energy pathways to be cleared, and the body to regain its innate balance. Emotions, beliefs, fears and sabotages that do not serve the individual cause energetic dysfunction and imbalance, which in turn results in a myriad of physical problems. Kinergetics clears the causes of dehydration. When the body is supported through balanced hydration, it is then able to access deep energetic imbalances that otherwise would remain hidden. Clearing stresses that block the assimilation of water opens the pathways for toxin removal, vitamin and mineral absorption, and lasting pain corrections. By accessing and clearing stress held in muscles, and especially the jaw muscles, Kinergetics has profound success with structural imbalances. The Kinergetics system addresses many physical symptoms from candida, allergies and pain, to learning difficulties and behavioural and motivation problems.

What It Can Help

Barbara developed glandular fever soon after receiving amalgam fillings. She presented with medically diagnosed Chronic Fatigue. Testing suggested mercury toxicity. After the hydration correction and having her kidneys energised, she was totally corrected, and her eczema also cleared.

Doctors were stumped with a lady admitted to hospital emergency in excruciating pain. Medical tests drew a blank. A Kinergetics student totally cleared her pain in two hours.

Ann was born with Rickets. After countless operations she was still in chronic pain and her foot splayed out 25 degrees. A few sessions later her pain was dramatically reduced and her foot was straight. Her foot was out because her jaw muscles were tight!

Joe had severe leg pain from a motorcycle accident and begged surgeons to amputate his leg. They refused. He came to a

Kinergetics consultant for sleep-walking which was corrected and as a bonus no longer has leg pain.

Jane took her usual B vitamins after a hydration balance and turned bright red. The redness was the niacin flush from suddenly assimilating B3. B vitamins and many others are water-soluble.

CLINICAL KINESIOLOOY

Clinical Kinesiology is a highly organized and complex system mainly used by health professionals, such as osteopaths and chiropractors. It was developed by Dr Alan Beardall DC, an American chiropractor. He observed that muscle testing was analogous to computer output, in so much as both are binary responses (off/on, strong/weak, open/closed), and could therefore be used not only to answer simple questions like which therapy to use by using therapy localization (page 16) but to collect information on more complex patterns.

Within this framework Dr Beardall developed sophisticated ways of working with the body as a bio-computer to access diagnostic and therapeutic information. From his discoveries he developed a number of techniques, many of which have been incorporated into other branches of kinesiology. Examples of these are finger modes, pause lock, and priority mode (page 49). Staying very much in the vein of computer language, a mode that represents a large complex of ideas is called a file. Another area pioneered by Beardall is the utilization of other reflex areas on the head and body. For example, points on the skull – cranial diagnostic points – represent different areas of the body, making it easier to find areas of dysfunction, while points along the Central meridian represent therapeutic entries which are often the starting point in many treatments.

It is a requirement of Clinical Kinesiology that all therapy reaches all parts of the body and this is checked by testing arm and leg length to see if they are equal. It is surprising how uneven these limbs can be at the beginning of the assessment. This procedure is always carried out at the beginning of a session and at the end for a 'before and after' comparison. Dr Beardall created his own range of nutritional supplements, called Core Level Products, to meet the need for proper function of each nutrient which included all the co-factors such as trace elements. Alan Beardall had discovered hundreds of finger modes and completed the majority part of this system before his untimely death in a car crash in 1988 whilst visiting England.

SELF-HELP FOR STRESS AND PAIN

Elizabeth and Hamilton Barhydt are the originators of simple self-help exercises to relieve learning disability, chronic pain and stress. Both have an extensive background training in kinesiology, combined with Hamilton's engineering background and Elizabeth's in psychology. They became involved with Touch for Health in 1980 and travelled around in their motor home sharing the information that they had learned. They found most people were not interested in taking a class, they wanted 'to be fixed now'. So the Barhydts found themselves doing more one-to-one sessions and developing simple kinesiology exercises for the people to use after they had moved on. Not having room in the motor home for a massage couch they developed techniques and balancing that could be done standing up. Their work, centred around retired people who were troubled by persistent physical pain and limited range of motion, led them to create an entire series of what they called basic balances. They published these in their book *Self-Help for Stress and Pain.*

Self-Help Approach and What it Can Help

neck and shoulder tension
limited range of movement
headaches
pains: shoulder (bursitis), arm (tennis elbow), wrist (carpal tunnel), knee, back
sinus pain and congestion
hiatus hernia
repetitive muscle stress injuries
jaw and ear ache
mental stress around learning
ear-eye-hand-brain co-ordination
neutralization of environmental stressors

This work is very effective with reactive muscles; basically, this means muscles that are functioning inappropriately in relation to others. Muscles work in groups to bring about movement and sometimes, especially through accidents, injuries or traumas, some muscles do not resume their normal state. The balancing procedures activate the mind/body intelligence through movement or touch which eliminates the need to identify specific muscles or reflex points. For physical pain you would move the painful area which tells the body this is what we are working on, carry out the correction, move the area again, and if pain remains repeat the procedure. Muscle testing is an option as you do not need to know which muscles are involved but just carry out the corrective exercises.

Sessions are both therapeutic and educational. After discussing the person's concerns and objectives for the session, the instructor/therapist will carry out a series of muscle tests using an indicator muscle to illustrate areas of imbalance. The person is then shown how to do the corrections on themselves. Participating in a workshop can bring dramatic changes as the following examples illustrate.

Case Studies

Whilst attending a weekend workshop in Bognor, one lady was able to discard her hearing aid in her left ear as the result of improvement. Next time she went for her hearing test her hearing had improved by 10 decibels and it is now almost normal. Muscle testing showed that she wasn't breathing properly. Age recession revealed that this was a result of having been party to a heated argument between her father and an aunt over the way he treated her and her mother. This happened at age four and she had been holding her breath for fifty-four years! Since that weekend workshop she has continued using the techniques successfully on herself. One success was being able to stop her right shoulder from seizing up which used to incapacitate her for weeks.

A lady had a pain in her thumb, especially when she went to start her car. This had been going on for six months and her doctor had suggested an operation to reduce the pain. Every time she tried to start the car she twisted her arm to activate the starter switch. So she was asked to twist her arm as she would do in this action and then do a reactive muscle balance and a frozen muscle balance plus working with the spindle cells in her forearm muscle. Within a few minutes she was able to go through the motion of starting her car without any pain in her thumb. After this she was able to start the car without any pain.

UK DEVELOPMENTS

The branches that have been described so far are the main developments in kinesiology which are taught and practised world wide. There are several UK based training systems in kinesiology, some of which are taught and practised exclusively in the UK. Readers can contact their kinesiology associations to keep them up to date with any parallel developments in their own countries.

Balanced Health

This is series of classes for lay people based on basic Applied Kinesiology taught by The Academy of Systematic Kinesiology which also offers courses to professional standard. The Academy was founded in 1985 by Brian Butler, who was instrumental in bringing Touch for Health to the UK in 1976. The Balanced Health curriculum covers all the basic tools of Applied Kinesiology and provides a sound foundation in the principle which practice of these skills. It teaches only the kinesiological procedures that are recognized by the International College of Applied Kinesiology. Emphasis is placed on a holistic approach which addresses all the four aspects of the human being, mental, chemical, physical and energetic. The practitioner will also look at life style issues, home life, work, food intake, sleep patterns and physical activities. A session could involve all the aspects previously described in Touch for Health and will include further advanced techniques from Applied Kinesiology.

The Academy of Systematic Kinesiology attracts to its training programmes a high number of professionally qualified participants and the following case histories are supplied by one of these.

Case Histories

Marie Cheshire is a registered nurse who has been working with kinesiology since the 1980s. Mrs A, aged forty-six, came to her suffering from ulcerative colitis, having had an ileostomy in 1986, which involves removing the entire colon and rectum. She was complaining of severe pre-menstrual tension, insomnia, food intolerances and was unable to handle stress. Treatment from her GP had not been effective. Marie Cheshire's treatment included identifying food intolerances and nutritional deficiencies (using Riddler's reflex points), dietary advice, working on the adrenals, using injury recall (cell memory of injuries) and techniques to improve her self-esteem. Within six weeks her pre-menstrual tension had disappeared and in five months she was completely symptom free.

Mrs B, aged thirty, suffered from agoraphobia for six and a half years after her father had died suddenly and her second child had been born prematurely. She had previously attended a stress clinic, received home visits from the health visitor and psychiatric nurse and was on anti-depressants, all of which had given her some benefit, but she was still unable to cope with being outside the home environment. Treatment consisted of emotional stress release, cross crawl, temporal tap, clearing past traumas, breathing, chakra and cranial corrections, correcting the ileocecal valve, Bach flowers and nutrition. She improved rapidly and by the end of the month organized a family reunion at Brands Hatch, the first time she had been able to tolerate such a public occasion since the onset of her illness. Since then she has continued to make steady improvement.

Creative Kinesiology

Creative Kinesiology was the inspiration of Haakon Lovell, an acupuncturist, who learned Clinical Kinesiology from Alan Beardall. This system concentrates on working with subtle energies to increase people's potential in life. Having created a system to work from, Haakon then taught his work to others. After running a year-long course in what was then called 'Energy Awareness' in 1989, he sat back exhausted and decided he didn't want to do that again. He then worked closely with Carrie Jost, an experienced kinesiologist and psychotherapist. Together they produced a training programme which is now known as Creative Kinesiology. The focus of Creative Kinesiology is subtle energies, meridians, what is the quality of the chi – the life force, chakras, the spiritual level, aura, etheric body, emotional body, mental body, astral body and the relationship and connection between these. It looks at ancestral influence, such as inherited attitudes or trauma, working with the person's blueprint and on the DNA to bring about changes through healing. It helps identify behavioural patterns, especially ones that are continuously being repeated.

Many clients who are looking for fundamental changes in their lives will see Carrie for several sessions over a period of months. Others are looking for help with a specific problem, as the following case history illustrates.

Mr Y was afraid of the dark. He was also afraid of blackness; the colour black made him fearful. Creative Kinesiology techniques traced this fear to his ancestral past. Carrie worked on his meridian energy and chakras to clear this ancestral influence. Further work touching points on his head lightly and also massaging points on his feet restored his energy and he felt much happier and stronger.

Cyberkinetics

One of the quantum leaps for kinesiology has come about through the work of Alan Sales, a UK research kinesiologist, who developed Cyberkinetics, a system which regards the human body as a living bio-computer. He has developed a new way of testing muscles which he calls analogue muscle monitoring. This unique procedure tests muscles dynamically as they move through their range of motion with the person resisting as the practitioner applies a constant pressure. When the muscle locks or shows any deviations from a smooth continuous pathway this information is referred to as the display of its analogue status which is then used as the basis to balance the stress in the circuits.

This new way of testing muscles combined with the discovery of the modality concept forms the backbone of Cyberkinetics. The modality protocol appears to allow the "body's innate intelligence" to go straight to the heart of the problem thereby directing the practitioner to the deepest underlying imbalance quickly and efficiently.

Cyberkinetics' maxim is to find the one single most important energetic correction which is needed to produce the most profound beneficial effect on the rest of the body.

Optimum Health Balance

Charles Benham first encountered kinesiology in the late 1970s and this system is the result of his own questioning and inquiring mind and his experiences when working on clients. The name Optimum Health Balance is derived from the notion that each one of us has an individual optimum health level that is the highest possible level of health which can be attained for us in a single treatment given all the circumstances in our life at that time. The object of a treatment session is that the person reaches that level at the end of the session. Charles describes his system as a bio-computer approach, based on pictorial symbols, finger/hand/body modes, verbal or written challenges and channelled energy healing. Remedies or supplements are placed on the person's body for their energy patterns to be channelled.

Muscle testing is carried out using muscles in the groups as they naturally function, this means testing both arms and both legs. Your muscle response will then be checked against a series of symbols on cards representing various health levels, such as Vital Energy, Physical Energy, and recorded in percentage terms. Treatment is given, followed by further checks to make sure the treatment has been sufficient and no further treatment is needed. Optimum Health Balance can be used effectively to help a wide range of problems as the following case history shows.

This case is notable for the fact that the problem proved highly resistant to treatment. A retired man in his sixties had suffered from severe and continuous sciatica pain in his left leg and buttock. Apart from this one problem he considered himself extremely fit and testing confirmed this. Initial treatment proved more effective than any of the others he had tried but after six sessions there was no further improvement, so it was suggested there was no point in continuing. The client, however, elected to carry on, saying that he had a strong feeling that it would work in time. Two sessions later the client woke pain-free. He has been going on long walks, a favourite pastime, and his sciatica has never returned.

reprogrammes the energy flow so the imbalance is less likely to recur. This therapy is based on the practitioner feeling and even seeing the energy blocks so that s/he is eventually able to move and clear the blocks through mental effort. The ultimate power of our minds and thoughts still remains to be fully explored. Many of us are aware of how visualization (seeing with your mind) has been used by a number of people to free themselves successfully from chronic illnesses. It is accepted that illness and disease show in our auras well before they manifest in the physical body.

8

Other Natural Therapies and Kinesiology

The doctor of the future will give no medicine but will interest his patients in the care of human frame, diet and in the cause and prevention of disease.

Thomas Edison

Just as Goodheart found all these different links, connections and reflexes that worked together, so kinesiology itself works well with many other natural therapies. Much of kinesiology's popularity lies in its ability to complement and support the practitioner's skills which is why so many other qualified therapists add it to their own discipline. Muscle testing as a biofeedback tool is invaluable.

ACUPUNCTURE

Kinesiology has its roots in acupuncture. Marek Ubanowicz, a traditionally trained acupuncturist with a long-standing involvement with kinesiology, has this to say about the relationship between the two:

> Applied Kinesiology has based its meridian theory on the Five Elements in a simplified form. There is no mention of the distinction between channel problems or organ imbalances, no inclusion of pulse qualities or major energy blocks and it does not look at deeper meridian pathways. In time some of this will be included, especially as more acupuncturists study AK.
>
> The contribution AK has made to acupuncture is that it has defused a therapy often talked about in poetic and abstract ways and shown that it can be validated in an accessible way through muscle testing.

Bikram Deal, a graduate of the College of Traditional Chinese Acupuncture and Systematic Kinesiology, has successfully combined the two therapies in his practice. When working on a client, he carries out evaluations using both systems with the aim of finding out what is impeding the person's natural healing abilities. When there is an overlap in the imbalances, kinesiology enables Bikram to decide which to deal with first.

A young woman in her twenties diagnosed as having ME initially responded well to acupuncture and then required structural corrections in her upper neck and lower back before she made any further improvement. These corrections were defined and corrected by Bikram Deal using kinesiology. Treatments were carried out over several months during which digestive disturbances, light headedness and dizzy spells disappeared. This young woman has now been without any ME symptoms for three years.

It was June Tranmer's enthusiasm for Touch for Health combined with a fascination for Chinese philosophy which led her to seek a way of helping people by training as an acupuncturist at the Northern College of Acupuncture in 1988. As the course progressed, June began to co-ordinate traditional Chinese medicine with Touch for Health balance, carrying out the appropriate treatment without needles until she graduated in 1990. June feels that she is in a unique position as an acupuncturist as she uses kinesiology at the beginning of every treatment. The following are cases where June has used kinesiology as the key to unlock the door to healing:

> Mrs J needed help for withdrawing from tranquillisers along with coping with the side effects and symptoms of withdrawal. After a year of working on various aspects with good results, the ileocecal value (valve between the large and small intestine) repeatedly showed as a priority through muscle testing. Correcting it helped her backache and digestive problems but the corrections did not hold. Further testing showed that Mrs J needed a candida remedy. Since then she has gone from strength to strength and feels 'like a normal person'.

> Mrs W, aged seventy-four came with a mixture of complaints; her main problem was her back but she also had problems with her digestion, knees, bladder and a long-standing emotional trauma which she didn't want to discuss in front of her husband who

always accompanied her. After about eighteen months things weren't changing much but she wanted to continue with the treatments as she felt better. Emotions finally came up one day as a priority when the husband wasn't in the room and after a session of emotional stress release Mrs W had complete relief from her back pain. There is still more work to be done but now the direction is clear and her other ailments are improving.

AROMATHERAPY

Aromatherapy uses essential oils therapeutically to treat a wide range of conditions as well as maintaining good health and promoting well-being. Robert Tisserand has included kinesiology in his training programme for aromatherapy for the last thirteen years. As it is part of the course from day one, Tisserand believes it is very important that students are aware of both the benefits and limitations of kinesiology. Kinesiology is not a panacea, it is a useful tool which can be used to help the aromatherapist select the appropriate oils. Being able to access the energy flow of the client through muscle testing further enhances the whole treatment.

BACH FLOWER REMEDIES

Dr Bach intended the flower remedies to be a simple self-help method that was available for everyone. The remedies treat the emotions, the personality traits and the temperament rather than physical complaints. They play a vital role in revealing stresses. Kinesiology can be used to find which essences are needed and sometimes they are the only treatment required as the following case illustrates.

A married lady in her fifties, who worked on a checkout in a food store, went to see Charles Benham with severe migraines which lasted two to three days and occurred every month, though not at a regular time within the month. These mainly affected the right side of her head and were accompanied by nausea, depression and a feeling of coldness. She had had the problem for ten years and tried various treatments including acupuncture and homoeopathy. She also stated she was allergic to citrus fruit and suffered from pain in her left hip and leg as a result of a car accident which had happened several years before.

Testing revealed a definite link between the migraine and allergic reaction; further testing showed a pelvic displacement on the left side of the body and 'active' scar tissue on the left leg. Treatment consisted of two Bach flower remedies, Clematis and Scleranthus, to be taken two drops of each in water four times daily for ten days. This was the only treatment required.

CHIROPRACTIC

Kinesiology came from chiropractic, which is a manipulative therapy that works on the spine and joints. One British chiropractor, Richard Cook, member of ICAK who cannot imagine his practice without Applied Kinesiology, writes:

> The main advantage is one can prioritize body problems and thereby key into the major areas that require attention. It does away with guesswork, the old 'pop and pray', and allows the practitioner to obtain better, faster and more predictable results, which is better for all concerned.

The following are two case histories:

A nine-year-old girl suffered from asthma, which had worsened after her parents divorced. Chiropractic treatment concentrated on mobilizing the rib cage and some cervical vertebrae (bones in the neck) adjustments. Kinesiology testing revealed a cranial problem, dural torque (twisted pelvis), poorly functioning immune system and a diaphragm imbalance. After five treatments she was off her inhaler, her colour had improved, energy levels increased and she was feeling much better.

Mrs P, aged thirty-eight, complained of weak and painful legs, tingling in the hands and had been diagnosed as having MS for sixteen years. Chiropractic per se is not of great value in the stabilization of MS, but working with kinesiology opens other avenues and much can be achieved. The patient exhibited a reaction to sugar, problem with her neck, dural torque and problems with the mercury amalgam in her fillings. Muscle testing showed a need for Bach flower remedies and Richard is working in conjunction with her dentist who is removing the offending fillings – in the order determined by muscle testing.

After six months of regular treatment her general health has improved along with her energy levels.

Isobel Stevenson, a McTimoney chiropractor, uses kinesiology prior to manipulation when emotions or nutrition show as a priority, as Isobel has found that any manipulation will hold better if these are resolved first. For structural imbalances Isobel will muscle test to find which specific adjustments are needed and in what order. Kinesiology enables the client to participate in their treatment and become more involved in their own healing.

COLOUR

Colour plays an integral role in our lives. It can evoke feelings, create a state of harmony, enhance our appearance, inspire, and help restore our health and well-being. We are constantly surrounded by colour even if we pay it little attention and it forms part of our expressive language: 'green with envy', 'yellow streak', 'red with anger', 'feeling blue', 'in the pink', 'black mood' and 'white as a sheet'. Colour can be used to help both physical and mental problems and is a therapy in its own right. Kinesiologists will use colour in their balancing when appropriate, by having the person visualize the colour, by placing the colour on the body, or by having the person look at colours whilst muscle testing to find which colour has a strengthening effect. Sometimes a colour may also be depleting the person and muscle testing will show this too.

Heather Willings, guided by intuition and mediation, has produced a series of coloured patterns as an aid to health. When the patterns were finished, there were twelve of them, which suggested there might be a connection with the twelve acupuncture meridians. By dowsing, Heather managed to correlate two of them and then showed them to friends without explaining what they represented. One lady with asthma was immediately attracted to the Lung pattern, another with circulation problems chose the Heart pattern. Further verification was needed: using muscle testing it was found that when someone was attracted to a particular pattern, the muscle associated with that meridian was invariably weak. Looking at the diagram for that meridian has a strengthening effect on the muscle.

One other wonderful way of utilizing colours is by choosing

colours to suit your skin tone and colouring and, although this cannot be classed as using colours therapeutically, the improvement when someone is wearing the 'right' colours is outstanding. What you see is a vibrant person. And for the person themselves the experience is uplifting; every little glance they have of themselves raises their energy level.

COUNSELLING

A kinesiologist doing emotional work would do all the work through muscle testing and kinesiology treatments. A traditional counsellor, on the other hand, would be involved in talking to the client and would not engage in any hands on work or energy work. Maggie la Tourelle, a holistic health care practitioner, uses kinesiology as an adjunct to counselling and finds this allows her to work as a counsellor but in an holistic way which she feels greatly benefits her clients. The following expresses how Maggie feels kinesiology supports and works with counselling:

> Mind and body are part of the same system and it is sometimes important to use kinesiology to test for and correct imbalances that are affecting the client's emotional state. For example, brain hemisphere imbalance can result in the client either being too logical and not being able to consider alternatives or, on the other hand, being irrational and not able to take things step by step. Kinesiology can test for brain hemisphere integration and correct imbalances with cross crawl exercises. Some clients can be over-focused – they seem to have blinkers on, and activating acupuncture points can help such clients take a wider view. Diet has an effect not only on body chemistry but also on emotions. Therefore finding and correcting any foods or drinks that are contributing to how the client is feeling will complete the picture and support the overall changes that they are making. Stress is often accompanied by muscle tension and pain. While dealing with the emotional issues in counselling, kinesiology energy balancing can release the tight muscles and relieve the tension. Kinesiology also offers specialized techniques which can be used as an adjunct to counselling for dealing with emotional conflict, phobias and addictions.
>
> Mr K was a thirty-five-year-old artist. He had a history of depression and difficulties coping with situations in his everyday life. He also suffered from back problems which had not improved

with orthodox treatment and this contributed to his depression. Counselling helped him to deal with his life better and to feel stronger but his back problem quickly dragged him down. Kinesiology treatment helped his back problem. He also learned to use the emotional stress release technique for himself and now feels he has more control over his life.

DENTISTRY

Brian Thornton, a conventionally trained dentist, had for twenty years dealt with dental phobias with sympathetic reassurance and as gentle a treatment as possible. It was through his wife's severe back pain that he was to discover a simple yet extremely effective way of helping people overcome their fears. Impressed by the results of just one session of Touch for Health, after which his wife was able to bend down and touch her toes for the first time in two years, Brian obtained a copy of the Touch for Health book. He found he could treat his wife's back himself through following the instructions in the book. Brian went on to become an instructor and during this time he came across Dr Roger Callahan's work with phobias. Since then he has worked extensively with fears and phobias using muscle testing and Callahan techniques (page 41).

A patient with a history of fainting and vomiting after dental injections thought he was allergic to the anaesthetic. Questioning revealed that the onset of fainting varied between two minutes and two hours after the injection. A truly allergic response time would have been much more consistent. The patient was treated for the simple phobia of injections. Two days later he returned for treatment of the abscessed tooth which had brought him for dental treatment in the first place. A test injection produced no allergic reaction and the treatment proceeded; the tooth proved to be only half dead and, as soon as the patient was aware of pain, he fainted, even though he was lying flat. When he regained consciousness, he was sick. Brian concluded he was phobic to a whole range of dental procedures. Further treatment using Callahan's phobia tap cleared all the patient's fears relating to dental treatments. He is now a relaxed and confident patient and a visit to the dentist no longer produces any adverse effects.

Richard Sudworth has used Applied Kinesiology in his practice over a number of years to expand his dentistry treatments to work with the whole person, a form of holistic dentistry. Richard uses kinesiology in his treatments especially if there are problems with nutrition or structure or the possibility of allergy to the mercury in amalgam filling – a topic which is now being given a considerable airing. Richard Sudworth writes:

> The relationship of the jaw joint to the rest of the skeleton cannot be emphasized enough. What goes on in the jaw joint is profoundly related to the structure and function of the neck and lower back. Kinesiology can assess and correct a wrongly positioned jaw joint and this is the only way of consistently and accurately finding the best physiological position which makes the patient feel and function better. This type of treatment is used with patients who complain of headaches, bizarre aches and pains, general lack of well-being and, most critically of all, those patients who feel they have been abandoned and labelled as malingerers. Kinesiology can be used to assess the suitability of treatment, nutritional support, various filling materials for teeth and so on.

HEALING

> Healing is the outward sign of a restoration to inner harmony and balance.
>
> Louis Proto

Laying on of hands, faith healing, psychic healing, spiritual healing, magnetic healing and, more recently, therapeutic touch all refer to the human potential for influencing or transmitting energies for healing. Accepting humans as energetic beings with a constant flow of energies both within and outside of their bodies enables us to understand how simple touch can help restore a person to health and well-being. Healing is the rebalancing of the subtle energy fields. There are many areas in which healing and kinesiology overlap although the latter may at times be working on a more physical level. Michael Mann, a healer with a background in Touch for Health, found that when working with neuro-vascular points in particular, he was channelling healing energies to the points needing to be balanced and achieving that balance within one or two seconds.

Maggie la Tourelle combines both healing and kinesiology. Many people are sceptical about healing and would not go to a healer for treatment but would come to a kinesiologist. By placing her hand in different places in the energy field whilst muscle testing and observing the muscle response, Maggie can identify imbalance in the aura. The advantage of kinesiology is that it actively involves the person in the process and this physical demonstration is often the first experience the person has of the presence of something s/he cannot see. This experience can help them connect with their own sensitivity; they may start to feel sensations such as cold, heat or tingling when hands are held near but not touching their body. Muscle testing can identify precisely where a problem is located, its distance from the body and what is needed to restore that energy field. Healing treatment may involve the therapist holding their hands in that area (which is often all that is needed) or colour, sound, flower remedies, gems to name but a few.

Kinesiology provides a wonderful vehicle for introducing health students to subtle energy work and healing. They discover in the first two days of their training that they can feel the energy in the meridians and can have an energizing effect on them. This is something they had previously thought only 'healers' could do. We all have the potential to be healers. It is a matter of where and how we focus our attention.

Mr N was suffering from depression following a family bereavement. He also had a recurrence of an old back problem which was so severe he could not work; he was extremely worried as he was self-employed. Kinesiology assessment identified which vertebrae of the spine were involved and gentle energy work, just holding the points involved, allowed his spine to align and released the pain. Exercises were given to help strengthen his back. Further testing revealed allergies that were undermining his system and contributing to his condition. His physical condition has greatly improved, he is back at work, and he is able to deal with his grief without the added physical problems.

HERBS

'Herbs are essential and extremely valuable for supporting, cleansing and strengthening an over-stressed mind and body, whilst deeper psychological issues are identified, worked on and cleared using kinesiology,' writes Marion Bielby, a medical herbalist. Marion finds that combining the two therapies facilitates our ability to self-heal more quickly and completely. Many people have multiple problems. Knowing where to start, which herbs will be most effective, in what combination and in what dosage – all can be ascertained with sensitive kinesiology. Because the person is involved in the whole sequence they can see for themselves what the issues are which enables them to make a deeper commitment to their own welfare and take more responsibility for their own health and well-being.

HOMOEOPATHY

Homoeopathy is the healing principle of treating like with like. It is based on the principle of a minute quantity of a substance being used to heal the same symptoms as a gross amount would produce if taken by a person. It also uses the premise that only the *energy* of the substance is used, so it is diluted many times.

Cilla Higley combines homoeopathy with kinesiology, which provides a quicker and more effective treatment. Difficulty sometimes arises when deciding how and when to use a remedy. Muscle testing and finger modes can provide the answers to which remedy is the best for this person when more than one remedy is indicated, what potency (how diluted) to use, how often the remedy needs to be taken and for how long, thus eliminating the guesswork and providing the body with what it needs to heal itself. Homoeopathic remedies can help speed up the healing process of other substances – Bach flowers, vitamins – and vice versa.

HYPNOTHERAPY

Christine Baldwin, a qualified hypnotherapist, has been using kinesiology in her practice for the last four years with impressive results: 'Kinesiology now forms the king-pin around which my other therapies revolve.' Christine routinely checks her clients with kinesiology having found that there is often a problem with prescribed drugs, allergies, candidiasis or lack of essential nutrients which needs to be addressed before working with the subconscious. Very often the emotional/psychological problems will clear without hypnotherapy. Kinesiology can help reveal underlying causes though these may not always be accepted by the client.

A young woman of thirty-two, who had suffered from panic attacks which started after a minor car accident, came for treatment. The first impression was that this was a straightforward case of working with hypnotherapy to eliminate the fear associated with the accident. However, this lady was also taking thyroxine for an under-active thyroid. Kinesiology testing showed that her thyroid was over-active so, with her doctor's consent, she reduced her thyroxine. She then attended sessions of hypnotherapy working on the car accident which proved successful, to the point that she could drive the children to school and felt better in herself. But the next lab test showed her thyroid levels to be low and she was persuaded to increase her thyroxine: the panicky feelings returned.

A forty-year-old woman was suffering from bloating, hot flushes, anxiety, smoking thirty cigarettes a day, guilty feelings, frigidity, poor sleep, severe phobia of frogs, fear of menopause and panic attacks. Her medical history revealed she had been anaemic, had had two terminations and two D & C's and several teeth extracted. First Christine worked to erase the painful memories around the operations and used emotional stress release and age recession to help the woman come to terms with her former bad marriage and divorce. Further sessions of hypnotherapy have helped with the anxiety and fears. She has stopped smoking and the phobia technique has released her fear of frogs.

Hypnotherapist Allan Oakman constantly combines the emotional stress release technique with hypnotherapy and has great success in changing patients' negative patterns into confidence and positive action. For people who have exam nerves he has made it part of the hypnotic suggestion that they hold their stress release points prior to the exams with good results.

GEOPATHIC STRESS

Additional threats to our health can come from abnormal or disturbed natural energy fields, generated by the Earth itself. Disturbances in these fields can be caused by mining deposits, underground streams, erection of buildings, underground transport systems, sewage pipes or high voltage cables. As we are beings of energy it follows that we can be affected by energy and it is not uncommon to find several people living in the same street or working in a particular part of an office block whose health is being affected by geopathic stress. There are a variety of methods available for neutralizing geopathic stress – iron and steel rods at specific points, placement of crystals, mirrors, water, metal sheets, harmonizers and a variety of patented devices. Each situation needs to be evaluated individually.

MASSAGE

Kinesiology blends very well with massage and gives the therapist extra skills to work with when easing tight muscles or aches and pains. There is no need to muscle test. One can just work on the relevant reflex points or trace the meridian pathways (page 30). Working down the spine gives an opportunity to stimulate all the neuro-lymphatic points situated there.

MUSIC

If several muscles are switched off, playing the right kind of music (Baroque, Bach, Vivaldi) can bring about a strengthening. John Diamond MD, a psychiatrist, traditional healer and author of several books, has been using music – traditional, classical and jazz – as a therapy for thirty years. Music is part of the rhythm of life and has the potential to raise life energy and enhance the function of the thymus gland. The opposite is equally true: many composers and much of today's music have a deadening effect on life energy. Diamond has, with the aid of muscle testing, systematically tested 30,000 musical recordings on students and developed an understanding of the kinds of stimuli that enhance life energy. Beethoven, Bach and Wagner are among the composers that he refers to as 'high energy' composers, meaning their music enhances the life energy of their listeners. The use of music as a therapy has led John Diamond to search for each person's personal harmony, his or her 'song of the soul' or cantillation.

NUTRITION

Both the following kinesiologists are highly skilled and work primarily with nutrition as they find this is what helps their clients most. They gather information by spending time talking to their clients and from a questionnaire sent prior to the first appointment.

In her work, Terry Larder uses a vast array of vials which contain foods, vitamins, minerals, herbs, amino-acids, homoeopathic remedies, Bach flowers, and gems tested as mentioned earlier by holding against the cheek. Much of Terry's work involves using a technique known as Polarity Reflex Analysis. This is another set of reflexes on the body which relate to nutrition/remedy needs for the different organs of the body. Polarity in this case relates to the direction in which the energy is flowing. Terry finds this technique helps her unravel complex health problems and home into the nutritional support and sets up the body to receive that support.

One lady with a really tight hamstring (muscle, back of the thighs) had been to several sports specialists who could only recommend stretching exercises which helped but weren't getting to the root of the problem. Through muscle testing, nutrition showed as a relevant area: sugar was the main culprit which was causing these muscles to tighten. Terry was able to demonstrate this by getting the lady to hold sugar between her lips and feeling for herself how the muscles tightened. Cutting sugar and coffee from her diet has eliminated the problem.

Another athlete who had been receiving conventional treatment for over five months for a badly damaged quadriceps muscle was found to have a bacterial infection. Terry gave him herbs with antiseptic properties and the problem cleared up very quickly.

Michael Kent uses kinesiology predominantly as a screening tool for looking at the nutritional status of the body, approaching most problems from the chemical angle, not because he thinks this is the answer to everything but because this is the way he works most effectively to help people. Nutrition is fundamental to our health: chemistry (the way the body digests and absorbs that nutrition) is equally important.

Once you've find the key to the problem, the response is so quick the body seems to be saying 'thank you very much, that is all I needed'. A woman came to see Michael Kent presenting only one symptom: every time she sat down she started to itch all over. There was no rash but it was extremely uncomfortable and getting worse. Allergy was a reasonable assumption but it didn't show; what did show was high blood sugar. She was given a nutrition programme to follow, the itching stopped just like that and hasn't returned.

A lady in her eighties with glaucoma whose peripheral vision was deteriorating rapidly was brought to Michael by her daughter. Kinesiology revealed a couple of key nutritional factors, for which he treated her. At her six-monthly check up, she had regained 50 per cent of her peripheral vision.

OSTEOPATHY

Clive Lindley-Jones is an osteopath who has integrated Applied Kinesiology with his work for a decade. He is also a trained counsellor and teaches Applied Kinesiology. He says:

> Increasing numbers of osteopaths are undertaking post-graduate education in AK. This is a natural and relatively easily integrated addition to osteopathic practice, as the basic tools of AK challenge and therapy localization enhance the skills of the osteopath. Many of the standard AK diagnostic tools are adaptations of original osteopath and chiropractic concepts, so that the introduction of AK into the osteopath's clinic can both enhance traditional skills in treating problems as well as expanding the diagnostic ability to more accurately treat the many functional health problems – such as food intolerance, candida, fatigue, hyperactivity, tempero-mandibular problems – commonly seen in osteopathic practice.

He cites two case studies where he has used Applied Kinesiology.

A twenty-seven-year-old engineer who had suffered from knee pains since the age of fourteen had been forced to give up rugby due to his painful knees. Assessment showed that he had a twisted pelvis and weakness in the quadriceps muscle on both legs. AK testing showed there were signalling errors between the muscles which attached to the knee and these were putting strain on the knee joint. The foot was also examined and found to have an imbalance in the bones. Finally, when all this was resolved, the quadriceps muscles – powerful muscles on the front of the leg – were still malfunctioning. When tested once no weakness was apparent; however, when tested in an aerobic repetitive manner they became weak after eight or nine repetitions. This kind of repetitive movement is just the kind of use walking or running induces. This pattern was corrected through treating the neuro-lymphatic points and nutrition. The knee pain was completely resolved.

Sarah, a three-year-old who had never slept properly since birth, had difficulty going to sleep and would invariably wake eight or nine times in the night. She also suffered from constant ear ache and swollen glands.

On examination, using a combination of AK testing and cranial osteopathic work, it became clear that several bones in her head were still under stress from her birth. After three treatments she was waking up only three or four times a night and did not wake herself up when she turned. AK was used to test for homoeopathic remedies which were prescribed and after six treatments Sarah was sleeping through the night and no longer suffering ear aches.

VISION IMPROVEMENT

Vision is important to all of us. If it becomes blurred, unclear, imbalanced, we want to do something about it. Natural vision is about seeing with every part of ourselves – eyes, feelings, dreams, inspirations, thoughts.

Anthony Attenborough combines the Bates Method with kinesiology which provides a more effective and comprehensive means for improving sight, relieving associated stress and maintaining healthy eyes. Sight is an instinctive function which needs to be provided with stress-free conditions to improve. Muscle testing can reveal unrealized stresses; these can then be balanced working with the body as a whole which results in the sight improving naturally.

Helen is a poor reader because her eyes don't work together. At the age of four she was given glasses to help with a squint which was later surgically corrected, the squint only presents now when she is tired. Helen stopped wearing glasses when she was fifteen. She finds night driving extremely difficult as she is sensitive to light and glare. Initially her eye movements were harmonized by using neuro-vascular points and her sight improved further by working on the underlying stress. Eventually night driving became the priority issue. Muscle testing revealed this as a stress which affected focus, brought up an early childhood experience and showed her to be allergic to light. The emotions involved were sarcasm, being overlooked and unloved. Age recession went back to ten days after birth when she was left alone in the dark. The emotions and this experience were rebalanced with kinesiology, stress around the issue cleared, and Helen was recommended to wear the colour green as a support to tolerating light, dark and glare. Five years have elapsed since her treatment and Helen continues to be confident when driving at night.

Conclusion

TAKING THINGS FURTHER

TRAINING IN APPLIED Kinesiology (pages 15–16) and Clinical Kinesiology (pages 88–89) is only available to professionals with a medical background whereas training in Touch for Health and the branches described in chapter 7 are open to everyone. Touch for Health covers many of the original Applied Kinesiology concepts, thus providing a sound basic training in kinesiology. It is a prerequisite for some but not all of the kinesiology branches. Contact addresses can be found at the back of this book.

I trust this book fulfils the aim of introducing you to kinesiology, what it is and how it works, and that you have gained a clearer understanding of how and why your body responds in different ways to your life style and the pressures put on it. In a book of this length it is not possible to cover any one area in depth; hopefully the 'tasters' will lead you to explore kinesiology further. Whether it be for seeking help for a health problem, as a self-help enhancement, or as a practitioner who wants to add to their skills or to gather more knowledge through reading other books or attending workshops, I wish you well with your journey.

Useful Addresses

KINESIOLOGY ORGANIZATIONS

CANADA

Health Kinesiology, Jimmy Scott, RR3 Hastings, Ontario KOL 1Y0. Tel: 705 696 3176

EUROPE

Applied Kinesiology Seminars, Eastcote House, Eastcote, Devizes, Wiltshire SN10 4PL, UK. Tel: 01380 813139.

ASK, 19 Westfield Lane, St Leonards on Sea, East Sussex TN37 7NE. Tel: 01424 753375.

Educational Kinesiology, Kay McCarroll, Body Balance UK Ltd, 12/14 Golders Rise, London NW4 2HR, UK. Tel: 0181 202 9747.

Health Kinesiology, Jane Thurnell Read, Sea View House, ong Rock, Penzance, Cornwall TR20 8JF. Tel: 01736 719030, Fax: 01736 719040, Email: info@healthk.co.uk, Web: www.healthk.co.uk.

ICAK Executive European, Thea Marshal, 54 East Street, Andover, Hampshire SP10 1ES, UK. Tel: 01264 339512.

International Kinesiology College Shifting, Sonnenstr. 15, Auslikon, CH-8331 Switzerland. Tel: 41 1 050 0588, Web: www.ikc.infro.com.

Classical Kinesiolgy Institute, Terry Larder, 81 Lancashire Street, Melton Road, Leicester LE4 7AF, UK. Tel: 01162 661962.

NEW ZEALAND

International College Professional Kinesiology Practice, PO Box 25, 162 St Heliers, Auckland, New Zealand. Tel: 00 64 9 574 0077, Fax: 0064 9 5570 8979, Email: office@icpkp.com, Web: www.icpkp.com.

USA

International College of Applied Kinesiology, 6405 Metcalf Avenue, Suite 503, Shawnee Mission, Kansas 66202. Tel: 001 913 384 5336, Fax: 001 913 432 1812.

Touch for Health Education, 6162 La Gloria Drive, Malibu, California 90265. Tel: 001 310 589 525269, Fax: 001 310589 5369, Web: www.touch4health.com.

Educational Kinesiology Foundation, PO Box 3396, Ventura, California 93006–3396. Tel: 805 658 7942.

Three-in-One Concepts, 2001 West Magnolia Boulevard, Burbank, California 91506. Tel: 0101 818 841 4786, Fax: 001 818 841 0007, Email: onebrain@earthlink.net.

Topping International Institute, 2505 Cedarwood Avenue, Suite 3, Bellingham, Washington 98225. Tel: 001 360 647 2703, Fax: 001 360 647 0164, Email: topping2@gte.net.

Self Help Stress and Pain, Elizabeth and Hap Barhydt, Loving Life, 1241 Ian Court, Sparks, Nevada 89434. Tel/Fax: 001775 358 1432, Email: feelgood@lovinglife.org, Web: www.lovinglife.org.

Advanced Kinesiology, Dr Sheldon Deal, 1001 North Swan Rd, Tucson, Arizona 85711. Tel: 602 373 7133.

Behavioural Kinesiology, The Diamond Centre, PO Box 381, South Salem, New York 10590.

BioKinesiology, John Barton, 1400 North Main Street, Cedar City, Utah 84720.

The Institute of Behavioural Kinesiology, Dr John Diamond, PO Drawer 37, Valley Cottage, New York 10989.

TOUCH FOR HEALTH ASSOCIATIONS

AUSTRALIA

Association of Australia, PO Box 4418, North Brighton, Victoria 3186. Tel: 003 9593 2077.

CANADA

Box 745508, Kitsilano Postal Unit, Vancouver, BC V6K 4P4. Tel: 001 604 978 6292.

EUROPE AND NEAR EAST

Kinesiology Association of Denmark, Hesteskoen 6st th, DK3000 Helsingor.

Touch for Health Association Holland, Groestraat 5151, Je Drunen, The Netherlands. Tel: 31 41637 5617.

Italian Touch for Health Association, Via Fili Bianchi 5, 25080 Maderno, S/G BS, Italy. 39 36 564 1553

Association of Systematic Kinesiology, 19 Westfield Lane, St Leonards on Sea, East Sussex TN37 7NE. Tel/Fax: 01424 753375.

Systematic Kinesiology, 39 Browns Road, Surbiton, Surrey KT5 8ST, UK. Tel: 0181 399 3215.

Kinesiology Federation, PO Box 17153, Edinburgh EH11 3WQ. Email: admin@kinesiologyfederation.org, Web: www.kinesiologyfederation.org.

Touch for Health Centre, PO Box 150, Bognor Regis, West Sussex PO21 2FN

SOUTH AFRICA

South African Association of Specialised Kinesiologists, 14 Osborne Road, Clarmont, Cape 7700. Tel: 27 21 61 8021.

USA

North American Touch for Health Association, PO Box 430009, Maplewood, Missouri 63143. Tel: 800 466 8342, 314 647 0115.

Touch for Health Association, 6955 Fernhill Drive DSte.2, Malibu, California 90265. Tel: 800 466-TFHA.

Further information on kinesiology training and addresses for the individual practitioners mentioned in this book may be obtained by sending a stamped, addressed envelope to the following address: Ann Holdway, 78 Castlewood Drive, Eltham, London SE9 1NG, UK.

Further Reading

Barhydt, Elizabeth & Hamilton, *Self Help for Stress & Pain* (Loving Life, Groveland, 1989).

Barhydt, Elizabeth & Hamilton, *Accurate Muscle Testing for Foods and Supplements* (Loving Life, Groveland, 1992).

Batmanghelidj, Dr F., *Your Body's Many Cries for Water* (Tagman Press, 2000).

Benham, Charles, *Optimum Health Balance* (OHB, 1991).

Blakley, Paul, *The Muscle Book* (Bibliotek Books, 1992).

Brennan, Barbara Ann, *Hands of Light* (Bantam Books, 1987).

Butler, Brian, *Kinesiology Balanced Health* (TASK Publications, 1990).

Butler, Brian, *Breast Care Manual* (TASK Publications, 1993).

Callahan, Roger, *Why Do I Eat When I am Not Hungry?* (Doubleday, 1991).

Campbell, Don, *The Mozart Effect* (Hodder & Stoughton, 1997).

Connelly, Diane, *Traditional Acupuncture, The Law of the 5 Elements* (The Centre For Traditional Acupuncture, 1979).

Deal, Sheldon, *New Life Through Nutrition* (New Life Publishing, 1974).

Dennison, Paul & Gail, *Edu-K For Kids* (Edu-Kinesthetics, 1987).

Dennison, Paul, *Switching On* (Edu-Kinesthetics, 1981).

Dewe, Dr Bruce & Joan, *Professional Kinesiology Practitioner* (Auckland, New Zealand, PKP Workshops, 1990–3).

Diamond, John, *Your Body Doesn't Lie* (Warner, 1980).

Diamond, John, *Life Energy* (Paragon House, 1990).

Edwards, Betty, *Drawing on the Right Side* (J. P. Teacher, 1979).

Fletcher, Susan, *What Can we Eat? What is Wheat Free?* (Merton Books, 1999).

Gerber, Dr Richard, *Vibrational Medicine* (Santa Fe Bear & Co, 1988).

Hay, Louise, *You Can Heal Your Life* (Eden Grove Editions, 1984).

Kendal, Florence Peterson & McCreary, Elizabeth Kendal, *Muscle Testing and Function*, 3rd edn. (Williams & Williams, 1983).

Krebs, Charles, *Revolutionary Way of Thinking*.

Kriegar, Dolores, *The Therapeutic Touch* (Prentice Hall Press, 1979).

Further Reading

La Tourelle, Maggie, *Thorsons Introductory Guide to Kinesiology* (Thorsons, 1992).

Mansfield, Peter, *The Bates Method* (MacDonald & Co., 1992).

Owen, Charles, *An Endocrine Interpretation of Chapman's Reflexes* (American Academy of Osteopathy, 1980).

Parker, Allan & Cutler-Stuart, Margaret, *Switch On Your Brain* (Hale & Iremongor Pty. Ltd., Australia, 1986).

Promislow, Sharon, *Making the Brain Body Connection Kinetic* (Publishing Corp, 1999).

Selve, Hans, *Stress with Distress* (New American Library Signet Book, 1975).

Stokes, Gordon & Whiteside, Daniel, *5 Element Rebalancing* (Touch for Health Foundation, 1981).

Stokes, Gordon & Whiteside, Daniel, *One Brain* (Three in One Concepts, 1984).

Thie, John, *Touch for Health* (TH Enterprises Publishers, 1973).

Thurnell Read, Jane, *Health Kinesiology* (2002).

Topping, Wayne, *Biokinetics Exercises* (Topping Institute, 1998).

Topping, Wayne, *Stress Release* (Topping Institute, 1985).

Topping, Wayne, *Success over Distress* (Topping Institute, 1991).

Walther, David, *Applied Kinesiology* (System DC Pueblo, 1981).

Westwater, Jan & Marshall, Bev, *Colour for Health* (Equilibrium, Australia, 1989).

Wirhed, Rolf, *Athletic Ability & the Anatomy of Motion* (Wolfe Medical Publications, 1984).

Index